CW00972936

THE
PSYCHOTIC
FIREMAN

"WELL, I NEVER EXPECTED THAT!"

MICK CROWE

Copyright © 2022 by Mick Crowe

Paperback: 978-1-63767-900-5
eBook: 978-1-63767-901-2
Library of Congress Control Number: 2022908582

All rights reserved. No part of this publication may be reproduced, distributed, or transmitted in any form or by any electronic or mechanical means, without the prior written permission of the publisher, except in the case of brief quotations embodied in critical reviews and certain other noncommercial uses permitted by copyright law.

This is a work of nonfiction.

Ordering Information:

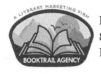

BookTrail Agency
8838 Sleepy Hollow Rd.
Kansas City, MO 64114

Printed in the United States of America

I dedicate this book to my wife and two daughters,
my friends, the young firefighter I walked past,
the NHS and especially my GP, who gave me space and time.

Table of Contents

INTRODUCTION

I need to write this book for future generations to learn from. If I were to do nothing, my experiences would be lost and I simply couldn't accept that.

My story covers a journey through the mind which occurred as a result of events in my life, but you need to realise what sort of person I was in order to understand the later parts of the book. It is a factual account of events in my life up until the day I decided to commit them to paper. You can analyse the information for yourself and draw your own conclusions as to what happened and how it has affected me.

The fact is, it is not easy to open up and share this type of information for fear of ridicule, victimisation and misinterpretation. But within these pages, you'll hear the truth, directly from the horse's mouth, so to speak, which I hope you will learn from.

I will tell you how I came to put pen to paper. Everyone I know is aware of a small part of this story: the fact that I was a fireman and that I fell ill. But most won't be aware that my illness is probably a mix of post-traumatic stress, psychotic depression and schizophrenia. I've never asked for a final diagnosis of my illness because what use is it to have a label?

I have nothing to hide and so I have no hang-ups about sharing deeply personal information with complete strangers via this book. I am sure it will surprise some of my friends, simply because very few know what I am about to reveal.

In the year 2000, I became seriously mentally ill. A few months later, I remember speaking to a colleague of mine, Peter, saying I'd lost blocks of time in my memory. In fact, I said, "I can't remember the last few months of my life," but I didn't realise at the time that it was far more serious. My memory had been completely gone for a while. I was in limbo and wasn't even aware of it.

As I came to understand the seriousness of my condition, I started writing down my thoughts and feelings in note fashion, as a coping mechanism. I compiled these for 17 years, but the strange thing is that as I look back, I can't even remember doing this. It's like I'm reading a book that relates to someone else. My mind simply cannot process all the information or the fact that what's written here is the story of my life.

As I started to read through my notes, I found that they didn't naturally fall into chapters. Thus, I needed to create some to try and get the book into some sort of format that hopefully you can follow. I didn't know what it would be about at first, but eventually a pattern emerged. It was a bloody hard book to write when you have my problems, so please bear with me and tolerate my English grammar.

As I sit in my man cave in the pavilion in my garden at the age of nearly sixty, I reflect that I once felt I had achieved everything I wanted to do by forty. Everything, except, for seeing my children, and hopefully grandchildren, grow-up. That sounds good, perhaps, but there was a flip side to it: my life as I knew it had, in my mind, already ended at forty.

I am about to embark on a journey, so come along for the ride. I will take you by the hand and gently lead you through my life story. Along the way, I will introduce you to realms of almost impossible experiences in my brain. You need not know it all, so I won't tell you everything. Some things remain locked away in the mind – the best place for them – hidden in a dark land that has no rules.

The book is finished but it will never be complete. What you need to know is on these pages, in black and white and I hope I have made it as simple as possible so it can be understood by all.

If I can get this right, I have a story to tell, a book the likes of which you have never read before. I can see the conclusion on the bottom of my pile over there on the table, but how long it will take until I reach the last page and whether it will all work the way I intend it to, I don't know.

Today is 1st July 2017 and I am attempting to sort my mind out on paper. It's quite a job, but please come with me as I delve deep into the fragments of my memory.

CHAPTER 1

Childhood

On 3rd of December 1960, the River Severn near Shrewsbury was at its highest ever recorded level and the midwife needed to cycle through floods to get to the Boathouse in Wroxeter. Water was lapping almost at the door's threshold, and inside my mother was in labour. I was born at about eleven at night and I screamed for the best part of six months. My mother told me later in life that I had, in her words, "driven her up the wall."

Home life was not good, which I suppose was perhaps because my father was raised in a Victorian-influenced way. He controlled us, hitting me, my mother and also my sister, who was seven years older than me. I remember my mother pushing her teeth back into position and holding them in place all night so they would set properly. I vividly recall the beatings and my sister being punched in the kidneys.

One evening while my mother tucked me into bed, I distinctly remember telling her I would throw my father in the river when I got older. I was about two years old and had only just started talking. My main concern at this tender age hadn't been asking to be read a story or for a glass of water before bed, it had been to comfort my mother.

I have vivid recollections of the Boathouse too. I remember a fox killing all our chickens, and my father threatening to cut off the kittens' heads with the shovel if we didn't leave them alone. But I also remember the games of hide and seek in amongst the trees and undergrowth. All the good and the bad times.

My family moved away from Wroxeter in the early sixties, when I was about three, to a new house on the outskirts of Shrewsbury, but things weren't much better there.

My mother was German and tried to leave my father and escape to Germany in the sixties, but this idea fell victim to red tape: she was alone in England with no family to help her, and my sister and I were British citizens. She was trapped.

She did manage to escape with my sister once, but my father, in a fit of authoritarian control, rang the police and they were waiting for them at Euston train station in London. When she did finally reach Germany, on her own, after tensions at home had escalated, I remember talking to her on the public pay phone with my sister and father beside me, asking her to come home again.

I never really knew my English family apart from my grandparents and two cousins and even with them, contact was minimal. My English grandparents were divorced and my grandfather was the main groundsman at the Roman settlement in Wroxeter in the sixties. Before that, he had moved with his family from a smallholding in Hope Valley, near Bishop's Castle, Shropshire, to take a job as Head Groundsman at the Atcham Airfield during the Second World War. Here, he was not only in charge of English workers, but also German prisoners of war.

I had some contact with my two English cousins, Bert and Mandy, in my early years in the sixties but lost contact with them until Bert fell ill many years later.

My mother worked hard to find the money to allow my sister and I to visit our family in Germany. She would hoe out sugar beet, work in the potato fields or as a cleaner to get the money for our train and ferry journeys. When I was older, I would often do the same sort of work at weekends or during school holidays, even though legally I was too young, because I knew the farmer. From the age of thirteen, I also had a paper round, but there was never enough money.

While he still lived with us, my father rarely let both of us children go to Germany with my mother for fear of us not returning. I believe it was emotional blackmail. Luckily, my parents separated when I was ten, which gave us respite. I was never happy with my father's behaviour and approach to life as I grew up. I learned right and wrong from my friends, and the relatives on my German side, whom I respected.

My visits to Germany exposed me to a massively different life to the one I lived in the Shropshire countryside. I stayed in Hamburg, a large city in the north of the country, and this showed me another side of life. Days there were mixed, with family visits and playing with my grandmother's next-door neighbour's kids in the sand pit. There was a girl, her older sister, and two older brothers. The girl was two years old, and I was nine, but as a child, age was far less important than who could build the biggest sandcastle. One of her older brothers, Karl, was my best friend, but I always had time for his little sister, pulling her around in a toy cart and tending to the various scrapes and knocks that she, as the littlest in our rough and tumble group, inevitably picked up. She was like my little sister, too. Little did I know that thirty years later we would be married.

One day, whilst in Germany, I had an unpleasant surprise in the elevator going up to my grandmother's flat. There was an older German woman in the lift alongside me and she verbally abused me just for being English. I was only nine years old at the time and I couldn't understand the aggression that ratcheted up, almost leading to a physical attack. Thankfully, the elevator door opened and I was able to escape before it did. When I was a kid, some of those who had fought in the second world war, or lost family and friends in it, turned against you, child or not. Isn't this world a dark place?

As I grew older and more aware, I often travelled to Germany only to find I was a "shit Englander" there and in England, a "fucking German". I was part of two worlds, but in the language of racism, that equates to worse than nothing. Some children in England were told by their parents not to associate with me because I was German. I was even victimised for my pronunciation – the terrible sin of having learnt English from my mother.

We lived in our second home until the turn of the decade when my father moved to Liverpool. He gave notice on the house in Shropshire while my mother and I were in Germany, expecting us to follow him. We didn't. Upon our return, my mother and I stayed with a friend until we were offered a two-bedroom flat. My sister had just left school at that time and had already moved out of our home, specifically to get away from my father.

Our new flat was in the same area as our second home. Times were extremely hard now and, although my sister tried to help, she was still only a kid herself. I gave my mother money from my farm work and paper round to help feed us, but while I received free school meals, my mother lived on egg and chips.

I was never usually troublesome as a boy, just what you would call normal. I'd been very close to my sister, even as a toddler. She would pull me out of the house in the middle of the night when my parents were arguing, and we would huddle up together to keep warm in the old barn across the road. Now, in my teenage years, she would discipline me to the extent of rubbing vegetables in my face for not eating them. It was annoying at the time, but we would be laughing about it by bedtime.

It was a massive blow to me when she died. I was only fifteen years old. Her sudden death from an aneurysm was a shock to everyone who knew her, but it was devastating for my mother, who changed afterwards and was never the same again.

I remember running to the public pay phone late one night, several months later, because my mother had taken an overdose of pills. I went with her in the ambulance and stayed there until they had pumped her out and she was stable. Once I knew she was safe and would eventually return home, I started on the seven-mile trek home in the early hours of the morning to an empty flat. I remember a doctor visiting her on her release, but there was no support from a mental health team or anything like that, and I was constantly worried she would do it again while I was at school.

That was when I really grew up. I no longer rebelled; I didn't have that luxury. I helped her as much as I could, and we got by, in the process becoming much closer. We were still struggling financially, but the odd pheasant or rabbit would find its way to the table to feed us. Our farmer friend, Kevin, brought most of them, but I shot and provided others. I didn't like the squealing if I got it wrong. In fact, I didn't enjoy killing at all, so I always either went for a head shot or let them run, knowing there would always be another animal and another chance for dinner. These kinds of animals were plentiful in Britain in the seventies.

As a result of being free from my father's clutches, we spent more time in Germany and even considered moving there.

Gleiwitzer Bogen in Jenfeld, Hamburg, had been a nice area in the late sixties, and it continued to grow during the seventies. This growth would lead to an influx of minorities, though, and by the late seventies it was renowned for its fights and gun crimes. A family friend was even murdered in his flat only a few storeys above where my grandmother lived.

I found it hard to get on with my German grandfather – he had no patience with kids. I remember being told by my mother of his World War II experiences. He'd been a young father at the start of the war but, by its end, he found himself in the midst of such traumas as collecting bodies off the streets after the bombing raids on Hamburg. He had a son, Herman, my mother's brother, who was drafted into the army at sixteen. Hitler had conscripted them all, from kids to ageing men, in the later part of the war. Even before being called up, he had, as part of the Hitler Youth, often been dragged from his house to witness deserters being shot at the barracks, learning the consequences of not obeying orders from a young age in Nazi Germany. After his enlistment, Herman was sent to the eastern front in Russia, only to be captured and sent to the Siberian salt mines as a prisoner of war.

A few years after the war Herman, was released from prison. There was no transport home, though, and so he did the only thing he could – hiked back from Siberia to Germany. When he finally made it back, his stomach was full of fluid from hunger and he was exhausted. All the food had to be hidden, since eating too much would have made him ill or perhaps even killed him. He had to eat slowly, my mother told me, to be able to return to full health.

Not long after his return, he emigrated to Australia. I met him on his return to Germany in the early seventies. There were problems between Herman and his wife and soon their marriage fell apart. With the benefit of hindsight, I would say he was probably suffering from depression. He was also drinking heavily, so it wasn't a good combination. Herman eventually took pills mixed with alcohol to commit suicide under a bush in a local park. We had searched for him all day, finally reporting him missing at about 8 pm. Herman's passing was my first experience of death, and I can remember my entire German family being distraught when the police found him. I was only twelve, drained after the day we had just had, sitting at the police station waiting for any news on my uncle. It was about 11 p.m. when they came to let us know he was dead, found in the very park where we had been searching for him earlier ...

Two years later, my mother's sister also died in hospital. With two of her siblings slipping off the gangplank so early in their lives, my mother was the last of her parents' three children still alive. This, along with my sister's death only a couple years later, and the fact that all my German relatives (apart from my grandmother and three cousins) seemed to die off relatively early in their lives, really knocked the stuffing out of me.

When I reached the age where I could get served in the pubs in Germany, I mostly drank in Jenfeld. That was when I met Helmut, a friend of the family who worked on the oil rigs in the North Sea. I enjoyed his company when he was back on leave. He was street wise, but obviously not as clever as I thought because he was the man murdered in his flat above my grandmother some years later.

As I got older and became more adventurous, I headed into the red-light district – the Reeperbahn St. Pauli. I was mixing with a man I'd met in a bar in Jenfeld, who was about my age. He had said he'd inherited money (he had a smart car so I believed him) and we got on well, playing dice and drinking like it was going out of fashion. He had a card for every club and I was offered anything I wanted, as long as he could watch me. That was my first sign something might be amiss and in the early hours of the morning, I found myself travelling to Lübeck for breakfast with him. **I woke up after a doze only to**

find him rubbing my balls while he was driving. I acted calmly to evade his advances, and directed him to a false address on my return to Hamburg, waving goodbye while pressing all the door alarms for the apartment building I had directed him to, hoping someone would let me in. I was lucky that someone did, and after he'd gone, I walked home. I was still young and quite inexperienced in life; maybe he was just acting out his fantasies or he was gay.

My mother looked worried when I told her the story, but my grandmother laughed and said I should have done a deal with him for what he wanted. She'd had a hard time during the war, as well as bringing up three kids, and she'd learned things the hard way. I guess, overall, she thought he deserved a feel of my balls since he had paid for most of the night out after I'd spent all my Deutschmarks.

"Any loving is good loving" is a phrase I've heard, and it's a phrase I agree with. While being gay isn't for me, I have many good friends who are and so I don't bear any grudges against the lad from that night out; we'd had fun.

It wasn't easy for gay people in my younger days. I remember a tale I heard in Liverpool during my teenage years, when I began to visit my father in Toxteth, Liverpool 8. A story about one lad being buggered with a broomstick because the other lads found out he was gay. That was about the time I heard another saying: "some hards are gay and some gays are hard". Come to think of it, I met no-one soft in Liverpool, but Toxteth was one of the roughest parts of the city. I heard a lot of stories there when I stayed for holidays, like how a live cat was thrown into the chip fryer at a local chippy one night.

I used to carry a lock knife everywhere I went when I was a kid; as a country lad, I needed one for whittling, building dens, tree houses, rafts, and skinning and gutting animals. I was very foolish carrying this through Liverpool because I didn't know how to use it as a weapon and I didn't want to; I was lucky I never ended up with it up my arse while carrying it. This same knife later became my work knife. In fact, I carried it for thirty years until my second visit to the psychiatrist where I handed it to him and simply said I don't need this anymore. The fact is, I had considered cutting a man's throat open with it a few years earlier in an attempt to carry out an emergency tracheotomy, something I will explain later. I'm sure I would have been locked up there and then if it had gone wrong; bloody hell, it was a stressful job.

Going back to my early years, I started primary school in the early sixties and did well in the first couple of classes with Mrs T. My achievement board was always full with gold stars. The headmaster, Mr M, was a bully and when I moved up to the junior class it got so bad that I eventually refused to go to school. He used to tie us to our chairs if we didn't sit still and bullied us verbally and physically. As a result, my parents moved me to another junior school, but the damage had been done by then – I wasn't interested in learning anymore. I enjoyed myself there though, and loved the nature walks. In fact, I have no bad memories of my time there, and eventually bought the school about thirty years later, converting it into a home for my young family.

I never sat my 11+ at junior school since my secondary school choice was the same, regardless of whether I passed or not. I wanted to go where my older friends had gone. I would never have applied myself to a grammar school education, so it wasn't such a bad decision after all; I was more interested in being a Tom Sawyer, building rafts on the river and tree houses or whatever. Later on, girls also came on the scene!

I suffered from bullying right from the start at secondary school. I soon learned to stand my ground with two individuals in particular, and, in fact, I gained respect in the school, even befriending my bullies, possibly because I had made life easier for them too. Even the hard nuts called me Mick now and life had become easier.

I learnt many lessons about life at school and not all of them academic. My most important one was never to break a promise. One day, my friend Arnold told me something and made me promise not to say anything. As it was, I did, and while it was something so insignificant to me, he was absolutely devastated. From that day on, I've never broken a promise. Years later, my psychiatrist asked me whether they could trust me; they wanted to release me from hospital and needed a guarantee. I just said: "Make me promise; I never break a promise."

Schooling was difficult and I flunked my exams in 1977. As you might have gathered, I didn't enjoy school, and my sister had only just died, so this was probably partly to blame. When I finished my education, I started an apprenticeship in bricklaying after turning one down as a car mechanic.

I found myself back in education at college doing extra curriculum work to catch up from my school days. I found bricklaying relatively easy and took to it quickly, but hated the winters, especially having to travel to and from work on a moped. I recall falling off three times in the snow one night. I passed my driving test at eighteen and bought a grey, hand- painted Mini Countryman with a bitumen roof. I was so grateful to have a car.

At that time, I joined my first real rock band which I played in for about eighteen months but found it was getting far too heavy for me and the enjoyment started to wane. It was a good time, though, but I'll go into these experiences later.

I finally had enough of my father by the beginning of the 1980s and ignored him for more than ten years. I had no contact with him until my wife pleaded with me to tell him he was a grandfather. As a result, he started to visit his grandchildren, but I wasn't happy. My wife eventually admitted she'd made a mistake and said she couldn't believe people like my father existed. Although my father has tried to make amends, especially in recent years, which has made things better, I still bear a lot of resentment towards him.

I was only earning £21 a week when I started working and would give my mother half of it since we still had no cash to spare. By the time I qualified as a 'brickie', I was earning about £55 per week, but the work situation was terrible. I put my name on the register to work in Germany since it was the *"Aufwiedersehen Pet"* days – if you remember the TV series.

I had finished my four-year apprenticeship and was doing my HNC in building construction – times were very tough in the building industry in that time. I had won the Silver Trowel and Challenge Shield for top apprentice and, at twenty-one, I represented the county in a national building competition in which I came sixth. I am sure this achievement was why I was kept on at the firm since people were being made redundant all the time. However, I then heard there were six jobs going at the fire service, so I applied for a job there, too. As it turned out, I stayed in England.

CHAPTER 2

Inauguration into Adulthood

My job with Shropshire Fire and Rescue service began in March 1982 after a rigorous selection process, as there were about 1100 applicants for six jobs. I always felt I must have been a little lucky to have been chosen, although I passed all the tests they had thrown at me.

To be completely honest, I think what I had accomplished in the building industry set me up for the fire service. I replicated my achievements there by winning the Silver Axe for top fireman recruit.

I'm not really a judgemental person at all, but soon after I joined the fire service, employment laws were introduced, and targets had to be met. The fact is, not everyone can be a firefighter: there was a rigorous selection process and many failed, some due to poor upper body strength which is essential in such a physically demanding job.

Unfortunately, during the latter part of my career, I witnessed many new recruits only just meeting the standards required and yet they were still hired in order to meet 'equality' targets. As a result, I had to watch as potentially brilliant firefighters were sent down the road. I hope things have changed now because I know what sort of person I'd like climbing through my window when my house is ablaze.

My first two weeks in the Shropshire Fire Rescue Service involved visits and lectures, and we were issued with kit. The six recruits from Shropshire ended up in Chorley, Lancashire, for a 13-week basic training course, followed by a 2-week breathing apparatus course before we were given posts on a front-line appliance somewhere in the county.

My first posting was in Red Watch, Wellington, Telford, and it was a real surprise just how hard I would have to work – both physically and mentally – to get up to standard. And that was only the beginning. There was still a probationary period of two years and a final exam after four if you had failed your Leading Fireman exam. Thankfully, I passed that relatively early in my career along with the sub-officer exam, so I didn't need to take it.

Our first day at training school was a different experience. We were ordered to get our hair cut that evening when the barber came, and there were talks on how we should conduct ourselves. There were also lectures on the venereal diseases which the local girls who latched on to the recruit firemen could pass on!

Kevin, Sam and Ray were my main pals at Chorley. Ray, an ex-commando; Sam, an ex-Merchant Navy Seaman; and Kevin who had had a variety of jobs in the Bridgnorth area.

Sam was a great character, a man's man, and his experience of sailing the seas shone through, even if we did rub up against each other a little at first. On the first day, he gave the barber his fifty pence and said, "Don't touch a fucking hair on my head, mate! I've paid you, now tick the register." He was as bright as a button, loved his dick and his drink, and was good to be around. I am still in touch with him to this day.

Ray, with his military experience, showed me a few tricks of the trade after I was bollocked by the instructor for having a dirty room. He told me I should clean the underside of my sink plug, wipe the bottom of the bin and the top of the doors and skirting boards, etc. Luckily, my bed pack was made perfectly, so it didn't end up outside the window like some of the others who had failed to meet his exacting standards. I have sadly lost touch with Ray over the years.

Kevin was my study partner. He was very conscientious and always worked hard. In fact, I should really thank him for winning me the Silver Axe award. Kevin would often ask me something, and if I didn't know it, I would find out from someone else and share the information with him. He pushed me even harder than I pushed myself, and I can genuinely say I would not have been disappointed had it been him who had won the course prize and not me.

The Shropshire lads stood out from the others and someone once heard an instructor saying, "Whoever picked the Shropshire lot certainly wanted firemen." As a result, we were always split up on the drill ground because, when we worked together, we stood out and were head and shoulders above most of the other crews. Kevin once had to run around the ring road that encircled the training camp in full fire kit because when he was told to give someone a hand, he had smiled and started clapping. It was not taken lightly by the instructors.

Most of our days were a fifty-fifty mix of theory and drill ground practical work. The instructors were hard men, with the good cop, bad cop who played off each other. An instructor called Potter was the worst – rather evil, in fact – and he was in charge of my squad. You couldn't get a worse type of instructor.

Potter worked us to the bone. I remember one blistering hot day sitting in the appliance as number two with my crew when he ordered us to slip the thirteen and a half metre ladder off the appliance. He made us run around the drill ground with it in our full fire kit and then replace it back onto the gantry before getting back on to the appliance. By the time he had finished with us, we were so knackered that this was almost an impossibility.

We couldn't believe it when he ordered us to do it again a few minutes later, but worse was to come. He commanded us to do it four or five times and, on the last drill, one lad dropped the ladder. Potter shouted, "If you do that again, you will do the drill over again." The lad was nearly ready to drop it again; we were going at a snail's pace now and Ray said, "Drop it again mate, and I'll fucking kill you." The lad dropped to the ground with the ladder on his lap, and he literally crawled with it on his knees.

None of us could hardly stand up, and my head in my helmet was pounding. I felt drunk, dizzy, sick and everything in between. I could hardly grip the ladder, but we somehow got back to the appliance. The problem then was lifting the ladder above our heads to put it back on the gantry.

Potter never said well done; instead he said, "It will never be as hard in the real world as it is here." As you will read later, that simply wasn't true.

On the positive side, we blokes had never been so fit – or at least, I hadn't!

One day the instructors put us Shropshire lads together on one exercise and we later found out they had put bets on us to win the drill. It took place on a tree-covered hill with a stream at the bottom and a water holding tank at the top for us to use in the event of the hill catching fire. The road was about three quarters of the way up the hill, with my crew at the bottom of the hill by the stream. We had to fill the tank from the stream below using only light portable pumps and hose, making a relay to the tank at the top.

At the end of the drill, we were ordered to take the equipment up the hill. The twist was the Shropshire lads were disadvantaged and had to carry the light portable pump from the very bottom by the stream up to the road, three quarters of the way up the hill to the truck. Other crews had to carry the other pumps up to the road, which wasn't as far because they had the advantage of intermediary pumps along the way.

When the whistle was blown to start the race, we were at the bottom of the hill behind every other team, but soon overtook them. We literally threw the pump over stone walls and steep banks to ensure it was on the flat-bed truck first, almost throwing it off the other side. We were good and fucking fit.

Other exercises and drills also tested us, such as the ring road where we ran in full fire kit with lengths of hose. Blokes would often collapse and had to be put in the recovery position and given water because of the heat.

The bungalow race was another one where each team had a ladder, hoses and other heavy equipment. The idea was to take everything with you through the inside of the first bungalow and then everything over the roof of the next bungalow then through the next again, until you reached the drill tower. Everything, including yourself, had to go up to the third storey of the drill tower. Next, the ladder and equipment were hauled up and put down the other side, then back to the bungalows to finish at the point where you had started. The twist was that whoever was last had to do it again.

Towards the end of the course it all became easier, but I developed hay fever for the first time in my life, so I struggled a little. People got hurt and left the job or were back-squadded to the next course to do it all over again. You just had to stick at it even with the steel in your boots wearing your skin off. The instructors became monotonous, screaming in our faces with the peaks of their caps touching our noses, but you could read them like a book after a while.

I always learned the hardest maths formulae and the sort of things that they were likely to ask. It was better than getting them wrong then having to carry a heavy piece of equipment around with you all week. If you were asked about a certain piece of equipment and got the answer wrong, you had to nurture it to the extent of even having to shit and sleep with it, but you never forgot it again. Luckily, I got away with that one.

The instructors would always pick on somebody. They broke many and they simply packed their kit bags and left. If you took the shit and handled it, they would always find someone weaker – it was the survival of the fittest.

When I was desperate during the physical drills, I would think of my dead sister – she was a strong girl and influenced me during my years as a teenager. She was like a ray of light among my darker days. I would often picture her and what she would have done and even envisaged her in the drill tower, beckoning me on: "Get that ladder and get up here!" I used mental tricks to survive it all, to keep me going, but I understood when blokes packed their bags and went home. To be honest, leaving never crossed my mind once.

One day, I came across a stray cat and her kittens, all bar one of which had been crushed to death by falling crates. Risking ridicule and discipline charges, I took the surviving kitten back to my room and nursed it. Before long, I noticed its pupils were different sizes, a sure sign of brain damage which I had remembered from first-aid lectures. My first room inspection after I had found the cat went well: not a single thing was wrong, even though the cupboard drawer was a cat's bed by the radiator. The instructor said nothing apart from, "Carry on, Crowe."

The simple fact was I was being trained to save lives and render humanitarian services – that would have been my response should they have said anything. None of the blokes ridiculed me; in fact, they would visit the kitten in my room, and I gained respect for looking after it. I received a bit of friendly abuse when I mercifully killed it on the fire ground, though, with the blokes hanging out their windows shouting "cat killer", but I couldn't let it suffer anymore: I did what I had to do.

We were made to crawl past large fires in the smoke room and to stand up halfway through. You could feel the heat in the upper part of the room and hear your hair sizzling and burning; we didn't need to be told to get back on the floor. Water was also sprayed on metal fires to show us how dangerous they could be. Magnesium explodes with a white light because it creates hydrogen gas, and I remember one recruit being burned on the neck by it.

Greg from Clwyd used to sweat profusely on a Monday morning, the beer from the weekend oozing from his pores while we were on the drill ground, but he never gave up. He was under pressure for his practical abilities so, in the evening, between duties, we would go to the garage and I would teach him what he was struggling with, even how to tie a bowline. I would explain and demonstrate while holding a line; knots and lines are something every firefighter needs to know.

In return, since he had been an accountant before joining the fire service, he taught me all the maths I needed to know. As a result, we both passed the training course with flying colours: he could now operate a pump and tie knots and lines, and I could do maths and understand equations.

People were weeded out of the course, even by fellow recruits. I remember one-night Harris was sorted by the ex- squaddies in his room because he signed us all in one hour late after a night out in the town. We could all have been disciplined with extra duties had he got away with it, but because I didn't trust him, I checked the register after he had signed it, and altered it to the correct time.

The end of the course was celebrated with one almighty piss-up; the stress that had built up over thirteen weeks basic training had to be released. The start of the evening also included drinking slops out of a bucket that contained fag butts and horse dung. It was a rough night and I was even thrown in a bath of cold water for winning the Silver Axe. Later that night, I ended up walking back to camp from the hospital, soaking wet, after escorting a Shropshire lad there in an ambulance after he had cut his arm open badly.

All we needed to do now was to complete our breathing apparatus course back at our brigade, and then we would be operational probationary firemen. At this point, I had never once given up on anything, but I didn't know what was ahead of me. It was the ultimate test of all time, which would be a matter of life and death, but that's something I will cover later on in this book.

All the Shropshire lads passed the course, and we were given our watch and station. Although not experienced enough to know exactly what lay ahead of us, we were now allowed to wear our epaulettes and call ourselves probationary firemen. We'd worked hard to get this far.

My initiation into the watch was to be black boot-polished around the balls and my knob chalked with pool cue chalk. It was all banter, and I didn't consider it bullying, although I witnessed some things which were out of order and stepped in to put a stop to them.

We played a lot of pranks on each other and laughed a lot, but many things had better not be aired. It was the eighties, and I'm sure anybody in the services or forces will know what I'm on about. Nobody wanted a bunch of 'pussies' coming to aid you in your moment of need; you needed to sort the men from the boys since your life might depend on it. It was a great time, though. Can you imagine a bunch of young men taking the piss out of each other, laughing in the face of adversity to quell the nerves? We had some nasty experiences at times and the humour and fun were a means of winding down, although I'm sure most of the public wouldn't understand it. These fun times are worth mentioning; it kept the moral and team spirits high. It formed a bond, a unit, but things were changing.

As I became older and one of the old hands, the younger lads would sumo wrestle with their pants pulled up the crack of their arses to see who could put who in a cold shower. In our free time, or stand-down periods, we would also play pranks on each other, setting traps with buckets of water over doors, jugging each other with water, placing crow bangers under the bed in a saucepan to scare each other, and countless other tricks – childish, you might think, but fifteen-hour night shifts were too long to be serious the whole time.

One evening, I remember the younger crew members throwing toilet rolls at each other's testicles, and the screams were hilarious. I walked through the dark dormitory later that night, and I assumed they were all sleeping or tending to their balls. However, once I'd passed by them, I heard Ned say: "Now that's what I call respect." I had to smile; I was a well-respected fireman, and it had its advantages being an old hand.

Tomfoolery was our speciality. We were once asked to paint a rectangle on the car park with 'officer-in-charge' (OIC) inside it for our boss to park in; we did it so small he had to park over it instead of in it. He went berserk with us, but we just cracked on daft.

Earlier on in my career, all the firefighters used to decorate the walls of the fire station when it was required until health and safety forbade it because of insurance reasons. Despite this, one day I painted Harry's smoking pipe as a prank, but he didn't take it too well; he came up behind me and poured the rest of the paint all over me. I didn't take it too well either, but we all had a bloody good laugh afterwards.

Harry had a short spell with mental health issues. He went to the doctor about his imaginary friend Barry and asked the doctor for another chair for him – this put him on light duties for some time. He also jumped out of bed in the dormitory one night, shouting: "Here's the window, Mick, let's get out!" before proceeding to climb out of the first-floor window. Ray jumped out of bed and raced over to pull him back inside since there was no ladder outside the window and we weren't on a job – Harry was sleepwalking.

When we were on jobs, we could see the funny side. We always acted professionally, but it was difficult on some occasions. For example, there was a time when a man's testicle had gone through and got caught in a plastic lattice chair and we tried to push his swollen ball back through the hole whence it had come. We couldn't help but laugh, trying to disguise it with coughing or whatever. I still don't think he should have tried to stand up since his ball bag looked like stretched bubble gum!

Most laughs were black humour in the face of adversity, like the day I turned over an old steel dustbin to climb through a burning mobile home window because the aluminium door had welded shut. As I stepped through the window, my foot slipped on glossy-backed magazines and got trapped under something. So there I am, one foot on the dustbin and the other stuck inside and my crotch on a hot aluminium window sill. Quite a predicament, to say the least. Then I realised my foot was trapped beneath a cooking human body, bubbling and spitting, and my natural reaction was to spray it with water. When the steam dispersed, and I wiped my mask, I saw it splitting open to show all the muscles and tendons, just like a sausage splitting open in the frying pan. Later, we had a good laugh about my misfortune.

Good things happened on the job, too. I once plucked an unhealthy looking kitten out of a pond from the bulrushes after walking out on a ladder laid flat across the span. Nobody claimed her, despite it being the front-page cover of the Shropshire Star newspaper that night, so I took her home and called her "Mosey" after Moses in the bulrushes, and she lived with me for a good twenty years. We went through the good and bad times together and were the best of mates.

CHAPTER 3

Living the Seventies, Eighties and Nineties

L ife was good between 1982 and 2000 apart from a couple of episodes. I suffered from stress in 1989 because of the job and I was never the same after this. However, it took me nearly thirty years to figure out what the problem was, but I can't go into the details for confidentiality reasons. It was a rather unique situation, and personal to me. Apart from that, I had an excellent job, a nice car and plenty of money. Everyone I knew was healthy, and I was even mortgage-free by the end of my late twenties.

Life changed for me after I joined the fire service; my money doubled and I became fully independent, taking on the tenancy of the flat where my mother and I both lived. She had married my new father-in-law, Rainer, who was also German, and moved out to go and live with him. I respected Rainer and had a lot of time for him; my mother was now settled with her new husband, and I was standing on my own two feet.

My mother took a back seat now, and I could do what I wanted knowing she was settled. I would still treat her, though, since she hadn't married into money. We'd had a hard life when I was growing up, even though she'd tried her best to provide for us.

I'd met my future stepfather Rainer in about 1980, not long before I joined the fire service. He had stayed in England after World War II when he was released from a German prisoner of war camp, and became a farm worker, although he was a qualified carpenter. He was the father I never had, and I thought the world of him. Rainer never spoke about the war back then, but he did say he was in Russia on the eastern front and had to escape from the Russians to be captured in the west because he feared for his life.

I took him to visit the Imperial War Museum in London and I was astounded by his knowledge of the war. After that, he shared many of his experiences with me, and I considered myself fortunate and privileged to be told about them and to have been born in a generation which hadn't faced major conflict in such a way.

He had spent time in the Luftwaffe, supporting the army, about one mile behind the front line. He was a corporal on an 88 mm anti-aircraft gun, but it was also anti-tank and personnel to support the ground troops.

When he first joined the air force, he was sent to France but not long after that he was sent to Russia where he found himself behind the front line, shelling the Russians over his own army. He was in the 'big freeze' where everything ground to a halt in minus 40-degree temperatures and trench warfare set in.

Rainer spoke about the waves of people coming out of the Russian trenches: the first wave would have weapons, the next waves picked up the weapons from the dead and carried anything they could find, including axes and knives, to attack the Germans. Even women would fight. They would be continually shelled, surviving by drinking the water from a nearby frozen pool only to find dead bodies rising to the surface in the thaw. I was overwhelmed by his stories; by God, he had seen a lot.

The retreat from Russia was just as harrowing. He explained how they broke out of the Russian military encirclement after eating horse meat to stay alive.

At the end of the war, Rainer escaped from a hospital train when he was captured by the enemy after taking a bullet to the thigh. He said it was easy to escape since most of the Russian soldiers were drunk. They were shooting any Germans wearing an officer's uniform; he himself was able to barter for his life because he was wearing a Luftwaffe uniform, being in the air force amongst what was mainly army personnel. He slipped out with two others after dark and headed west, to the British and Americans.

After arriving in the west, they were ordered to return to the east by the allied soldiers. But before they left, an English nurse tipped them off that a hospital train was leaving and heading further west that evening. That day, they hid and jumped on the train when it was about to pull out later that night.

Rainer and the other German prisoners of war were held in a camp in Belgium in the winter, with half a blanket each. I can't remember the exact figure, but out of about one hundred and twenty thousand soldiers, only about forty thousand survived. Money was provided to feed them, but it was pocketed by the allied senior officers and their food was made up from sweepings off the market floor and whatever was cheap to buy.

Isn't it funny there's no mention of this in history books? You often only hear history from the side of the victor, and not the atrocities which were committed on all sides.

I would often ask Rainer for advice and I'd take on board what he had to say. He was a wise man and I often thought he left me his guardian angel after he died. We became very close during the ten years up to his death in March 2001. He had a heart operation but complications occurred, so he had to go under the knife again. On the ward he was on, people were dying around him every day. I travelled around eighty miles a day to visit him between my shifts – once even in the heavy snow, using the hedgerows as a guide for the road. It often got too much for my mother, so I'd end up travelling alone.

I told him to keep fighting because I was going to take him home shortly. He said it wasn't that easy, but my answer was: "I've seen people give up and they died, and you've seen it in the war – you will get through it and I'm going to come every day to make sure you're fighting." I took him home two weeks later; I don't think he ever forgot the support I gave him.

However, Rainer only lasted another twelve months after my mother died, and I couldn't support him as I would have liked because by that time I was ill myself. I couldn't even sit with him when he died because I couldn't take any more death around me, but I'm sure he would have understood.

It was another eight years after joining the fire service before I got together with the girl with whom I'd played in the sand pit as a nipper.

During that time, I had a couple of girlfriends and I was a happy-go-lucky, carefree guy. I did a lot of partying and girls seemed to like a man in uniform, so it was an incredible time in my life. especially since I had a well-paid job, security, and was doing well at work.

As I mentioned earlier, I first met my future wife in 1969, after my grandparents had moved from Rahlstedt to Gleiwitzer Bogen, Jenfeld. The next-door neighbour had four children and she was the youngest.

At that time, our seven-year age difference didn't matter because I was great friends with her older brothers and sister too, and we played together whenever we could. I used to pull her around in a little cart which she loved; I can still picture her in her homemade shorts. Even back then, I loved her like a little sister. It was a whirlwind romance for me, even though it took another twenty-one years for us to get together and become a proper couple.

As I got into my late teens and twenties, my visits to Germany became less frequent, but I still enjoyed our encounters. I remember going over once to find out she had a boyfriend which broke my heart, but I consoled myself by thinking it was an almost impossible situation anyway.

We didn't get together until 1990 when I visited my grandmother again. I found out she was working and living away and her mother kindly phoned her so we could speak. I invited her over on holiday for two weeks, but we extended it to three as our relationship blossomed. That was the start of a two-year travelling relationship, going between the two countries – it was a fantastic time.

After my return from a long holiday in Australia in 1989, that came about after my first bout of stress, I had planned to emigrate. I put that on hold when we agreed she would move to England. Her spoken English was better than my German, plus I could hardly read or write her language, so it was the best decision. In 1994, we both holidayed in Australia together and even though emigration was discussed, we decided to stay in England and I gave up the dream.

My mother and wife tried to get on in the early 90s during the first few years we were together, but it soon went sour. Both of them were strong-minded ladies, but my mother was very possessive and simply wouldn't let me go, something which I'm sure stemmed from the early death of my sister. My mother could be a good laugh and loved her bingo, and I think she was happy with her simple life, but

I think she missed out a lot by not being close to her grandchildren in her later years because of this friction between both parties.

Music was always an enormous influence in my life, and I learned to play the guitar in my early teens. My mother listened to me and said she was sure I was tone deaf – she even said she didn't think I'd ever get in a band – but her comments just made me more determined. *Slender Thread* was the first band I joined in 1978; I had never played bass before, only a six-string guitar, but I was loaned a short scale Gibson. After two weeks, I'd learned all their original songs and a few covers and was playing in Liverpool city centre, in the Pyramid Club. Overnight, I became a local sensation – from nothing to as good as a local hero – and I couldn't believe my luck.

I played in the band for about eighteen months until our drummer, Jay, and I pulled the plug on the group. I had played many good venues and most major cities around the country during that time. But the music, although before its time, was getting far too heavy for me and I wanted something different. During all that time, though, we had supported Eric Bell (ex *Thin Lizzy*) and once had the possibility of supporting *Black Sabbath* because Jay was their drummer's nephew, but we never did.

I didn't play for another seven years until a band called *Temporarily Forever* (my second band) were looking for a drummer. I'd always been a frustrated drummer so I had a go and it worked out well. We then looked for another bass player; obviously I was not irreplaceable on the guitar... thanks, Mum! However, apart from a few gigs, we never got out of the rehearsal studio, mainly because of a personality clash between the singer and lead guitarist.

Naughty Moose was my last band, co-formed in 1992 at the fire station with Peter and Pat, two other firemen, and it became quite successful. The band name derived from the comedy series *Fawlty Towers* when the moose's head fell onto Basil Fawlty. We were given the name from our watch as they sometimes referred to Peter as "The Major", the character in the series. Pat introduced us to a lad called Joe, who became our rhythm guitarist/lead vocalist, and we played and travelled a lot, supporting talented bands along the way.

We then got to the semi-finals of a "Battle of the Bands" competition, things got serious and we needed to start signing contracts, and work through agencies. It was at that time that I had to decide whether to go professional or stay in the fire service, and the latter is what I opted for since my girl was now pregnant. Although I was a good solid drummer, I was never known for my speed or technical ability, and the music industry was a cutthroat environment. *Naughty Moose* folded in 1995.

Two years later, we had two lovely daughters. It was then that I bought my old school, which I had attended in the sixties, some thirty years earlier, and converted it into our home.

Life was challenging with two small children and, unfortunately, I believe we weren't natural parents, but we managed, and they turned out to be lovely girls. Two little blonde-haired angels. In fact, when they were toddlers, a friend of mine once asked me where I had hidden their angel wings!

I am just so sorry my illness deprived them of a father from the ages of three and five years right until now. But there was nothing I could do. I know it now and I always did, but I wasn't able to change how I was with my illness. Anyway, they were loved and cared for and I would still die for them. I've always tried my hardest to be a good father; here's a text I sent to my eldest daughter on her first night away at university:

Me:	*Let no man into thy kingdom unless he is worthy. Who wrote that then?*
Daughter:	*Was it Shakespeare?*
Me:	*No, I did, a minute ago! P.S. I put the condoms in the suitcase!*
Daughter:	*Study is where it's at for me, dad.*

Just like her mother, I thought, but at least I was realistic. Maybe I should have had boys!

After a long break from the building trade, I was laying bricks, blocks and putting a roof on again. It wasn't half as much fun as gigging around the counties, but I was happy knowing it was for my family. Things were tight converting the school into a home, but we dramatically increased the value of it and moved in in 1999 with our last pennies.

CHAPTER 4

Dark Side of The Fire

I had a brilliant mind until I fell ill; I'm sure I even had a photographic memory because I could picture incidents throughout my life as if they had only happened yesterday. However, when I fell ill, that all changed, and the last twenty years are a bit hit and miss. Now, certain memories are clear, whereas others are hazy or non-existent.

I've told you a little about the good and bad times in my life and in the job, but now I will go into the very bad times. Black humour, as I've illustrated, was rife and used to help us get through the tough days. It was a humour that probably would not be understood by the general public apart from those who have worked in similar environments.

I can still remember the first job I went to and also the first deaths I experienced. In fact, I faced six deaths in two days.

The first was a man who had hanged himself in the woods and I was selected to cut him down. I still clearly remember a poignant tear running down his cheek as I tied a bowline around him face-to-face.

The next night, I had a further five fatalities in a road traffic accident. It was a collision in the early hours of the morning, and it later transpired one driver with three passengers was playing chicken on the wrong side of the road. He'd been making other cars move over until a head-on smash occurred with a young man driving back from his girlfriend's. The 'chicken' driver had been drunk – it was a mess. I had to pick up one man, thrown out of the car, by holding his trousers and foot independently; he was smashed to pieces and his leg bent like a banana when I lifted it.

The following morning, Steve mentioned the man splitting open and all of his intestines spilling out over the road. I was puzzled since I couldn't remember it but at breakfast, a while later, I cut open a tinned tomato and the inside squirted out over the plate – I couldn't eat it. I guess I did see it, but I'd blocked it out. It took me twenty-eight years to figure out I'd been blocking out unpleasant experiences from day one in the fire service.

On another day, I was sent to stand in at Telford Central fire station until dinnertime. While I was only away for about three hours, my watch had attended a road traffic accident (RTA). A high-sided vehicle had blown over in a storm and landed on a car, crushing the two parents to death but leaving their two small children alive in the rear seats. The lads had to console them.

Spirits had been high when I had left work that morning, but I came back to a station full of silent men, lost in their own worlds. We sat down for lunch and nobody spoke a word to each other; everyone just ate and watched the one o'clock news on TV. It was only the cook and I who could see the change in the less experienced lads – they themselves didn't realise the effect the RTA had had on them. It was fucking sad.

I also remember speaking and cradling a woman in a car on a forty-five-degree embankment, while taking her weight off the seatbelt so she could breathe more easily. She told me her personal last wishes and I comforted her before her eyes eventually glazed over as she slowly died in my arms. I decided what she told me would die with her and I never repeated what she said.

It's not just what you see but the whole reality of it – the smells, screams, moans, pain, suffering and pleading… The whole fucking situation. Then you've got to go home after your shift and be normal again. But of course, not every job took its toll on you and much of the work was pretty mundane.

But I'm not going to sit here and write a catalogue of horrors; this book isn't about that. Yes, my life has been horrific at times, especially when I fell ill: imagine your worst nightmare and multiply it by ten.

All in all, I tried my hardest on the job. I wasn't perfect, much the same as any and every firefighter; we had all had the same training and worked as a team, but being young and learning from your mistakes is a must in any situation in life. I always told myself if anyone could do better, they would be wearing my fire tunic instead of me.

One regret I do have, which I still feel guilty about now, was a shift when I was on the emergency tender which carried all the specialist equipment for rescues. We were called out to aid an appliance at an RTA where a young woman had been burned to death. On arrival, we found she wasn't so badly trapped as to need our specialist equipment, so we were told we could return to the station. Whilst we were waiting, it transpired that she was a local girl with a young family at home, so some of the local blokes were rather upset. As I was about to leave the scene, I passed a young fireman I had not seen before and he was ashen, his face white, probably having witnessed his first fatality. He looked like a frightened rabbit in the headlights. He asked me how to go about getting the body out of the car and, with a nervous laugh, I simply replied: "With great fucking difficulty, mate," and just carried on walking, relieved to be going back to my home station.

Even today, twenty years later, I regret not stopping and talking to him. He was asking for help and was in shock, and I walked away and ignored him. All I had to do was speak with him. I wish I could have that moment back again; he was a casualty even though he was on our side. If that man ever recognises himself in reading this book, please accept my humble apology, but I was in shock too.

Although our training was good, it couldn't account for every eventuality. You had to be a jack of all trades and learn fast, often on the job, and when I started, we didn't even have mobile phones, let alone Google. If you had five firefighters on the truck, all with an average of ten years service, you had fifty years of experience on hand. Another life line was the ability to radio control room staff who would find any information for you as quickly as they could.

Things sometimes went wrong, like the day Joe and I nearly lost our lives and burned to death. There was a fire in the old Sankey Social Club building where all the windows and doors had been boarded up. I was number one in the breathing apparatus team and Joe number two. The fire was in the main hall at the centre or back of the building, where smoke could be seen rising from and spiralling through the roof. The main entrance was smashed open, and we were ordered into the passageway towards the fire, taking with us a 70 mm hose and branch.

We were being drawn along in what was a massive wind tunnel which fed the fire with oxygen. The noise was unbelievable and the force of the wind was making doors flutter as if they were made of balsa wood. I'd experienced nothing like it before: there was no smoke, and the colours and flames bursting through the roof were beautiful, licking everywhere, the crackling and roaring of the beast almost majestic.

Above all this commotion, we heard the officer-in-charge blow his evacuation whistle, which meant imminent danger and that we were to get out. Slowly, the wind tunnel quietened down and eased – this was the draw of the fire equalising in pressure, but the fire headed towards us, rolling and rumbling up the passageway. Joe was pulling me out backwards as I directed the jet and spray to the ceiling to stop the flames engulfing us and cutting off our exit.

Since Joe was looking at the exit and didn't realise our predicament, he shouted at me to drop the hose, but I knew I couldn't. Luckily, he dragged me out. Very quickly, the fire engulfed everything and the walls started to collapse. It was only then I could explain to him why I couldn't drop the hose. Just another day at the office – all of that risk just for an empty building.

I dare say I'm not the bravest man in the world, but I have got principles and morals. A brave man is not the man who goes in without fear. Bravado, 'yee-haaa' – that's all bullshit in my opinion. A brave man is the man who goes in knowing that if he didn't he would have to live with himself afterwards. If you go into a situation as the last man and do nothing, nothing more will be done, so then you have to live with it. True, I've made a few mistakes in my time, but I can live with the fact that I always tried my best.

What I didn't need was the treatment I received from some in senior management, particularly when I fell seriously ill in 2000. I was a strong-minded character, never rebellious but always stood my ground, and years later my work colleagues would tell me they never expected me, of all people, to develop a mental illness. It was not what I saw in the job, but the screaming and suffering; it fucked my head up, and at the same time we were being treated like second-class citizens by those in management.

I remember on one occasion several drivers, including myself, informed management that we thought the new appliances we'd just been given weren't handling correctly. They were checked over and deemed fit for purpose and put back on active service. Everyone accepted the decision – except me.

I filled in a FB 28 form, stating the rear ends of the appliances was like 'the tail wagging the dog' and I would continue to drive them at a reduced speed. Obviously, this was unacceptable and all the new appliances were taken off the run and the old appliances brought back. They then sent the new vehicles back to the manufacturer for tests and my head was on the chopping block!

At the end of the day, though, I was responsible for the crew I was carrying and the public on the streets, and I just wasn't happy with the vehicles at all. I felt they weren't up to standard. Eventually it was found that the shock-absorbers on the rear end of the appliances were the wrong fit and, on this occasion, the senior staff thanked me for my intervention on the matter. There were other times when I made my point and was probably considered a thorn in management's side, but hey, it was always for the right reasons.

Because a mental illness can't be as easily seen as a physical illness like a broken leg, I was treated like a fraudster. They perhaps thought I was just trying to get out of the job with my pension or maybe taking the piss? I had done my fair share of dealing with shitty jobs over the years and I didn't deserve to be treated like I was. I always got my hands dirty, but if I was not directly involved in the rescues, I would rarely wander over to see the carnage because I didn't need any more notches on my belt. I'd seen enough.

While on duty in January 2000, I had a phone call at work telling me my mother was in hospital, diagnosed with cancer and seriously ill. It took her six weeks to die with an aggressive tumour on her spine and during that time I could not comprehend why she had to suffer so much in controlled conditions. It wasn't as if she had been in an accident; circumstances were different and the hospital staff had all they needed at hand, unlike us on a job. When she died in February that year, I wrote the following:

Doctors did a shit job before her admission into the hospital and during her time there. The only one worth his salt was the specialist in Oswestry orthopaedic hospital. The doctor in Copthorne was an arrogant arsehole. Was the morphine driver broken, I asked myself? It didn't seem to operate fast enough by far. The hospice was brilliant though, and the people who worked there were angels.

My mother let out a long groan on her deathbed – her spine had broken, because it had deteriorated due to the cancer, when she had slipped off the toilet in hospital. It was the same groan as the severely burned man I had sprayed water on at a job four years earlier. It wrecked my head.

After signing off sick in late January or early February 2000, it took nearly twelve months before I was admitted to hospital. I still know the precise date: 18th December 2000. I never did blame any of the doctors, though.

I didn't know what the problem was and I couldn't talk to anyone about something I couldn't figure out myself. I started writing letters to the doctor and words flowed out of my mind but they were all mixed up.

This was enough for the doctor to send me to a psychiatrist. I had three doctor appointments with the GP, occupational health, and a psychiatrist on the day I tried to commit suicide; I'm afraid I had already turned the corner and felt I just couldn't live anymore.

Once I had been signed off sick, I totally blanked the fire service, including most of my colleagues. I needed total escape from the pressures of the job; my head was spinning with it. I turned to the bottle. My coping mechanism was avoidance of just about everyone who knew me and drowning in alcohol.

In the early stages of my illness, I found out that a senior officer had made remarks in an officers' meeting that he, too, could do with time off work due to stress and depression. This annoyed me and took my illness to a different level. The anger and aggression was so intense I could barely control them.

Looking back now, I can see why the doctor told me to get rid of my guns; I had twisted myself into the ground with frustration. I knew what I wanted to do, but I wasn't a soldier trained to kill, I was a fireman trained to save lives, so it was completely against the grain. It distorted my mind – my brain exploded and I'm still trying to tidy the mess up now.

After a few months of being ill, I was contacted to say my salary was to be halved which was normal procedure, but we could appeal to the Fire Authority to have my full pay extended. My union representative, Mike, attended the meeting with my wife, who represented me, because I was far too ill to attend. I was told by Mike that an officer from senior staff would also represent me. Eventually, I found out that all he did was give my name, rank, date I joined the job and the day I went sick. There was no character reference, background information or any opinion on whether I was a good or bad fireman.

The Fire Authority asked my wife if she could return to work to support the family – she told them I was not able to look after the children. She also told them I could not claim any benefits for her or the children since she had not claimed treaty rights. She could have, being from Germany, but she had not returned to work after our first child was born which created a problem, even though she had worked before and our second child came soon after the first.

The Fire Authority granted an extension of my full pay salary for another few months, but it eventually halved, even though occupational health had advised them I could be suffering from post-traumatic stress syndrome. This put me and my family under extreme financial pressure.

On the day of my suicide attempt, an armed response unit was called and retrieved me from the back of a bin lorry after the emergency button was pushed, the crusher only inches away from me. Once I was out of the crusher, police officers man-handled me across their car, handcuffed me and put me in the vehicle. Other officers checked on my family and my gun cabinet while I was taken to the police cells.

Whilst at the sergeant's desk, one officer wound me up continually, so I grabbed him. I could have seriously hurt him, along with maybe one or two others, but I didn't; I would probably have been given a good kicking from the others if I had. I reminded myself they were doing their job, in a fashion. The others were only puppies, young lads, while there was one arsehole whom I had no patience or time for… I was fighting for my life.

I was man-handled to the floor, hand-cuffed again and then piled into a cell for a long wait for my psychiatrist to arrive. Although it took around five of them to put me in the cell, I put up little resistance, but I do remember all of them trying to get out of the cell door at the same time when they released the handcuffs. What a day! After the psychiatrist interviewed me, he sectioned me under the Mental Health Act, and I was put in hospital.

I had disposed of my shot guns and license some time before my suicide attempt, on the instruction of my doctor. A friend of mine, Ivor, was a gun dealer and I knew I could trust him not to give me them back unless instructed by the GP.

After my wife visited the most senior officer in the brigade, he agreed to reinstate me to full pay. This was the first positive move the Fire Service had made towards us and I then remained on full pay until I retired in December 2001, just three months before my twenty-year medal for long service was to be awarded.

During my three and a half months in hospital, my health improved gradually. Whilst I was in the high dependency part of the hospital and totally out of my mind, my father caught one senior fire officer questioning me behind a closed door. This was despite being under twenty-four-hour surveillance, not meant to be out of sight, and certainly not questioned about the job. My father demanded they stopped because I was still not functioning correctly mentally and did not understand what they were asking me.

Eventually the Fire Service offered me support, and an office job, but I knew I couldn't even fulfil this role with my health the way it was. Don't forget, this would entail me working with the very people and job which had put me into hospital in the first place.

Although my doctors supported me by confirming I had a qualifying injury that would give me a little extra on top of my pension, the Fire Service fought it, causing me further stress. I finally won the case some years later with substantial help from the union.

It took me thirty-odd years to figure out a lot of things, and I still have flashbacks bringing fresh memories, adding more building blocks in my mind. I'm not cured and I never will be; I just hope I will continue to improve slowly, but there are many days I doubt that I will.

The world is three-dimensional, but I reckon I've spent a good part of my life in a fourth and fifth dimension. This is where I am going to take you to now and it's not going to be easy for you or me.

During my illness, I wrote three short stories, entitled: '3682 Words in a Nutshell', 'Puppy on a String', and 'One Stone in my Hand'. They all have a significance, and I hope I can show you why. I hope they will enlighten you about mental illness – my mental illness.

CHAPTER 5

Three Short Stories

Story One

3682 Words in a Nutshell

I've walked through the valley of death and lived in the land where the rules are that there are no fucking rules.

That is quite a broad statement, but it's taken me twenty years to get where I am now and I still fall into the dark times. I'm not out of the other side of my illness and I don't think I ever will be. I've got the battle scars under my skull to prove where I've been, it's just that they can't be seen.

Only the dark side can carry you through when the light side of you gives up. Winston Churchill called his depression his 'black dog', so I will refer to it as the black and white dog of my mind. My theory is when the white side of you collapses, the black one takes control and that is bad news; they should work together to rationalise your decisions and thoughts. You are tired all the time, but you still need to control that black dog. I could control it within reason – except for three really sticky moments which I've already mentioned.

This is not a statement of documented evidence, it's a description of my mental illness and the events which surrounded it.

My psychiatric report states a diagnosis can only be made after a passage of time, and I am still trying to find out what I am actually suffering from, and what is still holding me down.

Since my final breakdown, I have had great support from the NHS. However, I do feel there's a lack of support for the families of those who have a member who is affected by a mental illness, but that's a different issue, and not what I'm trying to discuss in this book.

I've never read a book on psychiatry or psychology, but maybe this will give you a little insight into mental health. Depending on your level of knowledge, what I write may be old hat. If that is the case, just disregard it.

My only sorrow while writing is that I physically destroyed such a lot of the information I managed to retrieve from my mind before I even went into hospital. It was as if it was never meant to be seen or heard – perhaps I didn't want people to think I was crazy.

Maybe after reading the following pages you just might understand what it's like being mentally ill and why it was enough to send somebody like me over the top. But what I write is only a fraction of what went on, bearing in mind I was suffering for ten months before I was finally admitted into hospital.

After a long incubation period, you end up on your knees in the doctor's surgery. You try to make sense of it all, but it's just a blur: you're confused and even more situations raise their ugly heads to hound you. The doctor sends you home and you try not to dwell on things. You try painting the house, but it isn't easy; not only are your hands shaking, but so is your body.

The kids scream and drop toys on the floor, noises which seem ten times louder than usual. Your wife nags you persistently, screaming, "What's the matter with you?", but it doesn't make any difference. The pub is the only choice left – fuck doing the painting – so you hang out with a few select friends. You become unkempt and don't give a shit about anything anymore.

Even when you sit on the toilet, your legs are shaking as though there's an electric current running through the seat and you know there's something seriously wrong. You go to bed to see if you can sleep, only to find when you are awake again that you're in exactly the same position as when you first dozed off. Eventually your wife makes up another bed in another room. She finally cracks and tells you she's going home to her mother for a few weeks because she's had enough. Little does she know that it's only the beginning!

Your basic instincts take over to keep you going: you eat, drink, sleep, shit, and that's about it. But you don't care. There's no feeling left inside you, and you don't give a fuck about anyone else. The strange thing is you love your family, but all you do is try to destroy the foundation of it. You even tell your wife to fuck off back to her mother's with the kids and stay there.

After months of destroying your life, a life which has taken a lifetime to build, you start seeing and hearing strange things. You find out that by closing your eyes you can see into your own mind. You can see where the problem is: it's in the back left-hand side of your brain in the form of a transparent bubble, but you dare not enter it. Its force is just too powerful. If you go up close, you can press on it and see things inside it. It's 'information', appearing to take the form of Turkish script, or like uniform, black match-sticks, ticking like a computer, which flicker speedily, like a digital stopwatch. You study this language and finally figure out an alphabet. Considering this is your own mind, you would think it would be easy, but in fact, it is one of the most difficult things you're ever likely to have to do.

This coincides with a period when you find it's possible to communicate by putting things down on paper, so you start writing letters to your GP. For the first time in months, you're able to communicate and escape from being a prisoner in your own mind. This is difficult because the information has to be translated in the front brain to write it three-dimensionally into English. In fact, you're in a trance writing it, as if you're not writing it at all, but another part of you is. Your hand just moves and goes with the flow; you're not even sure what will come out next. I am told it is called 'automated writing', something which comes from the depth of your soul.

There are three parts of the brain working, you are sure of it now, so it becomes other-dimensional. You have to press against it, read it, translate it, and move your arm and go with the feel more than anything else. You look at the information as if you're looking at a 3D picture to see the reality, but everything is the opposite.

After a while, you're sure you've tapped into a genius part of the brain, but you dare not enter it or let it take over. Its logic is outstanding, and it starts out by figuring out the following for you:

"How could you know you've lost your memory if you can't remember what you've have forgotten?"

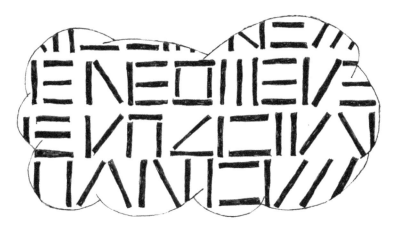

Alphabet

Or to put it another way:

"If you can't remember knowing something in the first place, how could you know you've forgotten it?"

Simple really, but when you're ill, it takes some figuring out, and I realised I had lost my memory. The brain is now starting to sort things out. In fact, it's starting to go into overdrive and will not let you sleep at all.

You visit the local hospital because the pain in your head is so extreme – especially the pain in your left ear. You think it must be an infection, or wax that needs sorting out. Everyone in the waiting room has injuries consistent with those you've seen during your fire service career. Not that you figure this out until much later, and you're convinced it was a set-up, when in fact it was a delusion.

During your wait, the burnt man you dealt with four years earlier sits down opposite you with a penetrating stare. It's so intense you need to cover your face to get away from it. Then you feel your head go on fire and blisters the size of bowling balls pop out of your cheeks and forehead. They were just like those you witnessed when you found a burnt body, bubbling and splitting open under your feet.

You then close your eyes to witness the inside of your brain like a central core jellyfish with millions of tentacles reaching to the extremities, quivering with energy. This is your brain coming alive again after a dormant period, after it has cut out for a while.

The light side is now kicking in, fighting to take over again. The dark and light sides of you battle it out to gain control. They bounce off each other, with the light side mainly in control. Then you regress; they become separate and don't work together, with the dark side becoming the dominant force. Luckily, the light side eventually wins because of your strong will. The fact is, you are so extremely ill, and nearly at the point of no return, that the chances of this happening are 50:50, and it's only in a split second that you actually turn to the light.

As a result, I made sense of the information from the depths of my mind. My left-hand earache was telling me the problem was what I had heard.

The severely burned man I had once helped by spraying water on him let out a long groan: it was the same sound my mother had made on her deathbed. I was also listening to my pump 'screaming' with my left ear, which I was responsible for, to provide water for the men in the building. I also had a lot of other things on my mind. It was a stressful job. Even now, my previous sentence requires great effort to put together since it's still mixed up in my mind.

I thought it was over and my problem was sorted. I don't know what happened, but I couldn't stay on top of it. I was so tired, I went under again, and things just kept getting worse. I became delusional.

You travel home one day in the car with your wife and see the farmers unloading straw from the lorry. They all wave, you now know you've got two choices: Make hay while the sun shines, or wave goodbye to life.

Things happened, everything you read or heard now had to be translated for you to understand it. Your wife is now going nuts at you. Years later, she tells you she would shake when you walked in the room.

You are convinced your mother is controlling your thoughts to encourage you to split from your wife. You just don't understand why your wife screams at you when you bring the wheelie bin in the lounge and start unloading it on the floor to look for something.

Probably a message you had written down from within your mind which you think you might need.

Around this time, you smell burning flesh. It's on the towels you wipe your face with. You find breathing difficult, so you cough in the toilet and are sick through heaving. You believe you're choking on the deaths of the many poor people you've seen suffer – and *you* suffer their pain; I did, so many times. Your body burns all over, such that you need to take off your shoes and socks to cool your feet because they feel as if you are walking on hot embers, like you've experienced many times.

You have a pain in your throat, which you relate to that of the man with the burned head who you once helped. You believe you are suffering his pain, and because you can now smell cancer all around, you're convinced you have throat cancer.

Your wife has another go at you and the aggression builds as she screams at you, watching *Saving Private Ryan* with the volume up. You lock in on all the gruesome shots, thinking about how realistic they make it look and the confusion of it all. You then totally reject the film and are convinced you are turning into a monster with your aggression, so you resort to dictating out of a book, to keep your mind clear, and after a while you doodle on the writing pad.

Oh my God, you think, *it's a pair of eyes with 'Mick, Mick, Mick.'* But what it is telling me is: three sixes – 6, 6, 6 – the sign of the beast.

You're now convinced you're going mad and work hard on controlling it. If you can't, you will just have to kill yourself before it gets out of hand.

You break down. You totally reject anything violent and shrink within yourself. Even the sight of a stray dog makes you want to cry because it has no home or food. You stare at the news and just can't believe you live in this world anymore. Why does life have to be so cruel?

Even when you walk past workmen in the street, jack hammering the road, you need to avoid it because the aggressive noises of the hammer on the tarmac are too much to bear. You cringe at loud noises and then realise you are far too sensitive for this violent world.

You know you have had enough when you even put the holly branches your wife asked you to cut off the bush for Christmas decorations in water. It is a real living branch, screaming out in thirst while slowly dying.

The experience starts slowly, without you knowing what is happening. The fact that you want to kill yourself is not because you can't cope with life, but the fact you have no option left.

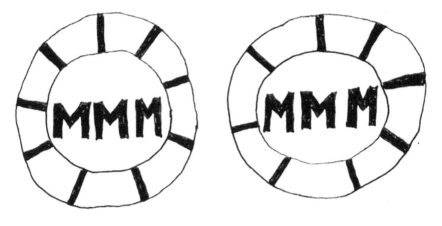

Eyes

To enter the other dimensions, as I call them, you need to be able to tap into that part of the mind at will, to find out the depths of your problems. The deeper you enter, the harder it is for you to find your way out. It is a very complex part of the brain, and although medication assists you in this, it is only the brain which can sort itself out.

The best explanation of this is that it is like a room full of filing cabinets but the files are not in a pile on the floor – they're all filed in the wrong place. Some cabinets are locked and you have to figure out how to open them without the number combination you need. Clues are hidden around the room to aid you, but you can't start sorting the files out until you look into the locked cabinets for other clues. Various clues are in the files you can see but because they are in the wrong order, you just can't find the one you're looking for. Every time you sort a cabinet room out, it shows you two doors. From those two doors and from the information you've sorted out, you need to make your choice and decide which one to go through. To be successful, you must go through this door into another filing cabinet room and start all over again. This goes on through a sequence of rooms, again and again, but if you pick the wrong door, you are back in the room you started with. Obviously, you have made a mistake somewhere and need to start over. Again, that is mental illness in its worst form– the files are in a total mess in your head. Nobody can help you with this. You are on your own.

But you do have some form of help, be it the clues given to you by the real world or the subconscious and the medication given to you. Your most powerful asset is your logic and intelligence, and by using that part of your brain you didn't know existed. This part of the brain is best left alone because it is so intense and beyond your abilities to analyse or understand. If you could understand how to use it, it would be greatly beneficial to the human race, but to me, as an average man, I couldn't begin to know how to control it back then. I believe I can now, to a certain extent, and maybe a deeply intelligent man could control it with ease. However, I believe the more intelligent you are, the more you want to look inside and then the further away it is to find your way out. But this could make you insane and unable to return.

This part of the brain is so unbelievable, and enriched with power, colour, smells and sights which don't compare to this world, and has a sinister side. To gain entry, you need to make this final sacrifice because it will never be experienced by anyone else apart from those who go in and accept its consequences.

The messages become stronger now as I can communicate with this dimension through **song on the radio**, *so I ask more questions*:

> *Where are we going to go?*
> **We're gonna go up high, high, high into the sky.**
> *But where?*
> **You're going to Jamaica.**

Did he say: "You're going to Jamaica" or "You're gonna meet ya maker"?

By this time, you've gathered enough information. After days of talking to the other dimension, you're ready to be 'one of the selected ones' to possess this supreme intelligence. But then something is stopping you!

You're told to come. The stars in the sky have a significance. The colours red, blue and yellow also have a meaning, but why? I need to find out why.

It is time to negotiate. I will not leave my family. They tell me my family can come too, but how will they live in this dimension? I tell 'them' I do not want to mess with my family so I decide not to go, because I love them and will not leave them. The messages from the voices then become sinister and I need to turn the radio off to stop them trying to take me over.

If I agree with the voices, they are supportive. If I defy them, they become angry. "I'm not coming!"

Don't mess with me boy, or you'll be sorry! You've crossed me – don't forget you're alone!

Now, things are all negative. I'm given the choice that I either come, or they'll take my family. You alter sentences around to find out what is really being said. You can't understand normal everyday conversation anymore because everything is mixed up.

The doctor says to you: "You will get better."

You ask yourself what he really said. Was it:

"You're ill, get better"?

"You better get well"?

"You better get ill"?

"Get ill, get better"?

"You better get your will."?

You are now convinced he's told you to get your will ready, or at least that's what your confused mind has understood. The doctor then asks how many pills you've got left.

You tell him: "X amount."

He says: "Well, that's enough for now."

But did he mean: "That's enough, four now."?

So, should I take four now instead of my original dose?

You calculate if you have enough to take four a day until you see him next – and you have! But what if you've misunderstood him?

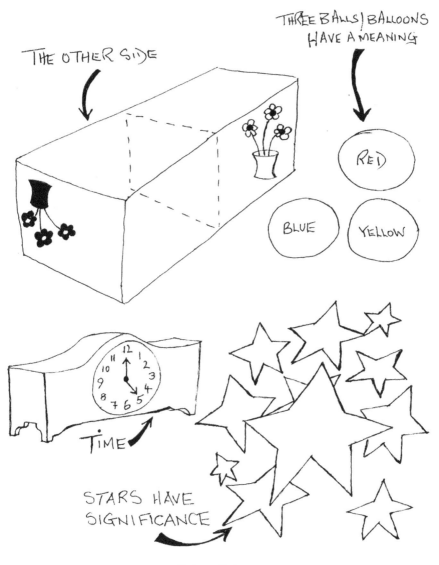

THE OTHER SIDE

THREE BALLS/BALLOONS
HAVE A MEANING

RED

BLUE   YELLOW

TIME

STARS HAVE
SIGNIFICANCE

Prime Colours

The day of the final solution comes near and you're convinced you're being cowardly by not wanting to leave your wife and children. You think the 'other dimensions' have arranged for your departure into death and the police will assist this dimension – the voices – to dispose of you.

You ask your wife if she wants you to go, and she says yes (she meant for me to pick the Christmas tree up). I'm now convinced she knows I have to go, to save her and the children. She has now lost all respect for me, knowing I'm putting them in danger.

You are now convinced an unsavoury group of men, employed by the other dimensions, are waiting for you in the porch. You don't want to open the door to them. How will they do it? Probably a bullet in the back of the head. Then an unmarked grave somewhere. You open the door and see no- one. Maybe they've given you one more chance?

You collect a load of pills and take a few bottles of beer to swig them down in a country lane somewhere, but your plan is foiled. The bin wagon is outside, and it is now I understand their logic.

The words 'face down in the crusher' come to mind. It makes sense; I'm not even going to get a burial. I'm just going to be pushed out of the back with all the rubbish and bulldozed into the rubbish dump. Nobody will ever know what happened and there will be no questions asked.

You're now handcuffed by the armed police and put into the back of the police car. Everyone's annoyed with you because you failed and they had to get you out of the crusher.

You're now convinced your family would have to suffer beatings and your wife raped repeatedly until your death, as punishment for making things difficult. It even crosses your mind your family will be murdered by them. *Thank God you took the guns out of the house,* you think; they would probably use them on your family, frame you and lock you up in a mental hospital for life.

In the jail cell, you make it easy for them by hanging your head over the toilet and covering the back of your head with a cushion from off the bed. *Just come in and blast my brains down the shit-house*, you think. But nobody comes.

You are now convinced they will drag it out and let you know that every minute you live, your family is being tortured and raped. You now know how they will do it: they will slowly burn you to death with propane so you suffer and smell the stench. They will even have a doctor standing by to keep you alive as long as possible with transfusions. You even wonder if it will be your own doctors. You even accept that's how it will be now.

Your eyes then search the room to get out of the mess you've caused. If you can kill yourself, your family's torture will be over. You spot a plastic cup the police gave you tea in and figure you can rip a slither of plastic out of its side with your teeth, pierce it into your wrist and then bleed it down the toilet, flushing the water. Even though there's a spy hole above the toilet, they never bothered coming in when I had my head over it.

The cell door opens. Your psychiatrist has turned up.

Once in hospital, you can't remember anything for days or weeks, but you slowly recognise yourself coming out of a kind of drunken stupor. You are told you had lots of visitors, but you don't remember any of them. Very slowly you get better and they tell you that you were walking on the tables and kicking the locked doors when the fire alarm went off, trying to give first-aid to an injured patient who fell over. You were paranoid, saying the nurses were trying to poison you and they were waiting outside to get you. Injections were given because you spat out the medication.

What a relief it is to see and recognise your family after the first suicide attempts.

IT'S ENOUGH TO MAKE YOU CRY.

Even though my wife was at her wits' end with me, she rallied around me. She was sick of the person I had become. Things I did, such as throwing the dishes in the sink from a distance, kicking doors open or demanding to go home when we were out because I didn't want to be there. She feared my mood, uncertain of what I would do next, and how I became aggressive after drinking.

She had to make my decisions for me because I couldn't fend for myself. Years later, she said she actually hated me but I had nobody else and she stood by me. She supported me one hundred percent after my hospitalisation.

Story Two

Puppy on a String

One summer's morning, a mother took her puppies onto the beach to a little cove known as Tranquillity Bay.

The puppies played cheerfully, as puppies do, jumping onto each other and giving each other playful bites. Eventually, they all wandered into the gently lapping waves of the sea to cool themselves off, away from the lovely summer sun.

Jet black shadows then appeared under the ripples of the calm water, moving directly towards the playful puppies. Not one of the little yelpers noticed a thing.

The attackers were both hungry and vicious, savagely tearing and ripping the puppies apart. Some puppies were thrown out of the water in the onslaught, with the slashing of a fin or tail, only to land in deeper water where they struggled and drowned.

Without a fight, the disembowelled puppies quickly hung suspended in the water, like puppets on a string, the occasional limb flinching with each tug.

The mother was desperate, running towards the sea, hoping her puppies would come to her. She started whining, yapping and pawing at the edge of the water. At that moment, the largest shadow turned directly towards the beach.

As the shallower waters parted, a head appeared above the surface, creating a wave. It was an animal which developed ears, then a snout, a tail, and then four legs: a wolf. The mother turned and scampered up the sand to a cascade of rocks, jumping from one to another. Eventually, she stopped, not being able to continue anymore. She turned to face her aggressor, showing her teeth with a snarl, and hoping to gain enough breath to kill her enemy.

They faced each other, one on the rock, the other on the sand. The wolf turned and looked back towards the water, feeling insecure without his pack. He ran back to the water's edge, occasionally looking back at the dog snarling on the rock.

As the wolf entered the water, his legs slowly shortened and turned into fins, his ears withdrew and his tail triangulated, before he slithered back beneath the ripples and disappeared from sight.

On the south side of the bay, an onlooker had seen all this unfold, sitting on a high protruding rock near the water's edge. In a crouched position, he slid a couple feet down the sloping rock and then sprung onto the sand. As he did so, he lost his balance, fell forward and cushioned his fall with his hands.

Unperturbed, he got up, stood tall, clapping his hands together to remove the sand. Unbelievable, he thought to himself, *I've never seen a dog so aggressive before.*

Quite a story my mind had conjured, and while it was vivid, it took me a number of years to figure out what *Puppy on a String* was all about.

As I see it, the sharks were the fire service management; the puppies were the firefighters, and the mother was me – an old hand in the job. Her reaction was how I felt I had been treated. Read the story again and you will understand what I mean!

It really shows how I could no longer return to work as a frontline firefighter because of my psychosis and I certainly could not work with people in an office which had finally pushed me too far. I just could never again associate with certain people in senior management again.

I was retired within a few months of coming out of hospital and had to approach my psychiatrist for a report as further evidence to receive my pension. It still took a further four years for the fire service to agree that my qualifying injury should provide me with a little bit of extra cash, and that was after they had been threatened with legal action by the union.

The brigade fought me; they would not admit it was job- related even though all my doctors supported me. It was clear they just wanted to save themselves money, and even though I knew that to management I was just a payroll number, it just proved it even more.

My exit from the job was disgraceful, especially when I heard how someone with a serious health problem in senior management was dealt with upon his retirement. I don't bear a grudge against him, though, and in fact I worked with him when he was still a fireman and considered him a good lad. His illness was terminal, but my treatment compared to his was appalling.

Upon winning the pay enhancement from the service, the Fire Brigade Union asked me to write an article on my experience for their magazine which I gladly did. But when I asked my ex-colleagues what they thought of it, they said they had not seen it. Hence, I suspected the magazine had not been distributed around the brigade.

I called it *In the twilight zone,* which you will find on page 74.

Story Three

One Stone in My Hand

As I walked along the long, white corridor, I felt nothing. There was an incredible silence.

I had looked in each room behind the white doors to the left and right of me along my journey, and on each occasion had been given an answer to the question I had.

Becoming impatient now, I needed to know much more, and much more quickly. I passed many of these doors with the prime objective of passing through the double doors right ahead of me and into the bright light of the sunshine.

As I walked, a man appeared – though from where, I do not know! I recognised his face, which was full of sincerity and character. It compelled me to stop. He held out his hand and, in response, I placed my hand in his and shook it.

He had a German accent and asked me where I was heading at the speed of light and whether I had time to spare for a little old man because he needed to speak with me. I nodded my head and smiled, walking through the open door to my left, even though I had not seen him pass through it.

Once I was inside, I looked around and saw nothing. There were no walls, floors, nor doors – except for the one behind me. It was just one mass of white space, bar the little old man I had spoken to, who was now working on calculations on a white blackboard with white chalk.

"Where are we?" I asked.

"Well, what do you see?" he questioned me.

I thought for a second, confused at his response, and said, "Well, everything is white, including you, except for your complexion. Yet

I can see you with the white blackboard amongst the vast dazzle of white. How can this be?"

The old man smiled and continued to write on the white blackboard. He answered me in the form of a question.

"If you were to see ten white colours all the same shade on a white background and put them into a kaleidoscope, would you see the one white pattern or a pattern of ten whites?"

I pondered for a while before responding. "Well, you wouldn't see anything at all, would you?"

"Well, that's no surprise with your eyes," he said. "You just have to use a different perception! Think about it for a moment."

He left me standing there, deep in my thoughts for a while, the sound of his chalk scribbling the only sound to fill the surrounding air until I spoke.

"Well," I started.

"Well," he repeated.

"I suppose if you looked at ten different whites on a white background you would see nothing, but if they moved about you might just see a pattern."

"How do you work that out, then?" he asked.

"Because of the different shades of shadows thrown by the light," I said.

Silence deafened the room as the old man stopped his writing. "So I'm wrong then?"

"I didn't say that, did I?"

"Sometimes you can find an answer to a question which has never been asked. So, then you have to work out what the question is in order to relay it to other people. In turn, they will then know how to ask the question, and therefore you can give them the answer," he explained.

"I think I follow you," I answered, though confusion was still visible in my features. "But maybe the ten whites are insignificant. Maybe the question doesn't need to be asked – has it got any relevance to anything? Do we need to know about ten white shades in a kaleidoscope?"

"The problem is this," he said. "I know the answer to a question which has never been thought of or asked, so now I need to work out how to ask the question. By doing that, I can also prove my theory. I've been working on it since the early part of the twentieth century, and I won't let it go until I've solved it. This is the answer to everything."

"Good God," I said. "It's 2005 now, that's about a hundred years on one problem! Don't you think it's time to move on? Is it really worth it? You seem to need an answer more than I do. It makes me wonder why you're trying to help me."

"Wait a minute," he said. "Along this passage, it's whatever time you want it to be. I move up and down it frequently, do you understand?"

I walked up to the white blackboard and pointing to some writing said, "Explain this formula to me in layman's terms." He slowly went through it like a teacher to his pupil.

"Let me start from the beginning. The answer is in the mathematics. If $3x - 7 = 5$, we know that $x = 4$. As you can see, we have the answer before we know the question."

After a considerably lengthy lesson, I figured out for the first time that mathematics is just a different language or way of thinking. If it could be developed into a language, it would multiply the brain. It is a way of communicating where words can't be used. If we could speak mathematics, or something like it, we could converse ten times quicker and be deadly accurate in what we say. We might even give the other person an answer before they have even asked the question.

As we talked, we occasionally smiled at my limited knowledge and built up quite a friendship. We worked from his answer all the way back to the beginning. He looked at me for inspiration and I shrugged my shoulders and smiled.

"I understand what you're on about, but my mathematics isn't good enough to help you out here."

We both smiled and let it be. Then, I looked at him and spoke again.

"People who study the universe collect data to analyse and work on, but the answers come from their minds. So, are they studying the workings of the universe or the mind?"

The old man nodded approvingly.

"Now you're thinking." His expression then turned serious. "I am here to help you; there has been quite a discussion about you. In fact, some people at the bottom of the corridor have suggested you should never come back down. They thought it best to leave you to walk up the passage to the double doors and into the light. Few people get this far up the corridor with a return ticket."

"What do you mean by that?" I asked.

"Well, let's say you have come to the 'turnaround point'. Consider you are swimming through an underwater tunnel and can hold your breath for five minutes. When you reach two minutes and have still not reached the other end, you must decide if you should keep going or turn back. Since you are tired, it will take you more effort and time to swim back than it took to get to where you are now. This is your 'turnaround time'. You still have a chance to get back if you go now, but go any further, the oxygen starvation could render you brain damaged. If you continue, you will reach the other end like all the others do, and you will take your first breath in a New World."

Silence fell while I considered his words.

"I'm still a little uncertain about all of this," I said.

He understood and continued.

"Well, there are those from where you have come from who are pushing you up the corridor because you know too much – they don't want you to come back. On the other side, there are those at the top of the corridor who want you to continue for your own well-being."

I looked at the old man and said, "I think I know what you're getting at. Tell me more!"

"Well, you haven't fulfilled the entire criteria to continue ahead so you will leave something physical behind, and I'm afraid it needs you, or else it will walk aimlessly around without you. Luckily, most of those at the top don't think it's right for you to be in this position and want you to go back down the corridor and end this journey, at least for the time being."

My eyes stayed focused on him.

"I somehow feel as if you know what's just happened to me," I said.

"Yes, I do," he confirmed. "You are in a dangerous position and it was because of the way you responded to it that we insisted on helping you. I think you know there are far superior 'people' around from where you have come from who are either exploited and used by major governments, as I was, or locked up in mental institutions, unable to cope."

I spoke again. "Well, you know they contacted me. I agreed to enlist with them and I was promised everything I ever wanted, or will want."

"Yes, I know," he said. "But didn't it turn sour and vicious?"

"When I told them as long as my ability was never to be used in warfare?"

"You said it, boy."

The old man then approached me and we shook hands, then with his free hand he enveloped our grasp.

"I'm afraid you will have to learn to cope with the information you have gathered behind these closed doors," he said. With his two hands, he rolled my fingers into a fist and I could feel he had placed an object in my palm. I closed my eyes to hear.

"Mr Crowe… Mr Crowe… Mr Crowe."

I opened my eyes to see a nurse standing over me with a smile on her face while I slowly regained my faculties.

"You are German," I said. "I can hear a slight accent."

"I am half German," she responded. "How are you feeling, my dear?"

"As if I've been to hell and back."

"Well, you have been very ill. We even thought we'd lost you at one point, but you're recovering now," she said. She then picked up a clipboard from the end of the bed and wrote on it.

"What are you doing?" I asked.

"Oh, just writing some details for the doctor. I see he wants you to drink plenty of water – at least two litres a day, Mick."

"Can I see it?"

"Of course, my dear." She walked from the end of the bed and handed it to me.

I could see a graph, probably my temperature and blood pressure, and a note written underneath by the doctor.

Dr E. MC=2 Ltrs H^2O Min 24/7. Interesting, I thought, I think it means:

Dr E. Mr Crowe must have a minimum of two litres of water
in twenty-four hours, seven days a week.

"The doctor will be pleased with your progress. He spent a great deal of time with you. Shall I fetch him?" the nurse said.

I thought for a moment before responding. "Let him be, he's probably got a load on his mind."

The nurse nodded. "Anyway, what was that you had in your hand when I passed you the chart?" she asked.

I pondered for a moment, looking down at the sheets and lifting my hand, without removing my head from the pillow.

"I've got one stone in my hand. How would you say that in German?"

"Easy. Ich habe einen Stein in meiner Hand," she said.

I was silent for a moment.

"But I still can't believe it."

"Neither do I," she agreed. "It looks like a diamond! You've got a diamond in your hand." Again, silence between us. "Anyway Mr Crowe, why did you try to harm yourself in this way?"

"I didn't, I was attacked," I explained.

"Don't worry, you'll be okay. You've had a tough experience, but we know how to help you keep on top of it!"

I felt relieved.

"Thank God for that. I thought I was on my own!"

Key Phrases

One stone

I recognised his face

German accent

constantly

speed of light

This is the answer to everything

exploited and used by major government

German

I can hear a slight accent

I am half German

I've been to hell and back

E.MC=2

Time

einen Stein

Albeit

Conclusion E = mc², but it's not the answer to everything.

E. MC=2 Ltrs H²O Min 24/7; Time travel is not physically possible yet (H2O = physical matter). Then again, you could say… is it all in the mind?

SHORT STORY SUMMARIES

Well, if you thought story one and story two were complex, then I can imagine you weren't prepared for an even more difficult experience in *One Stone in My Hand*. For the last story, I took you by the hand and led you through the mind.

The reason I say led, and not showed, is because it is a bit of a puzzle and you will have to figure it out yourselves. With stories one and two you were given some background information, but in story three you need to refer to my 'A4' and 'A2' equations (see pages 78 and 80). Read them together, but first I will give you some guidance on how to read the equations.

Quite some time ago, I drew a yellow star with a question mark in the centre of an A4 piece of paper. I didn't know why I had drawn it; as I said earlier, sometimes my brain leads my hand and I don't know what's coming out next. As I started working away from the star and question mark, an equation formed and it kept on developing right across a much larger A2 sheet of paper.

It is a moving equation – sometimes I move information, take it out, or add something new. What you have just read is just one stage of this developing equation, which might be totally different now since it is an ongoing piece of work.

When you look at the A2 piece of paper, you could say it's an equation of my mind, but it is also the chapters of my book. I can't sort my mind or my book out until I have got it into a logical order, which means I'm a bit of a mess at the moment.

At the time of writing this, I'm at a T-junction in my mind and I can't figure out which way I should go – left, or right. I'm still struggling to figure out the answer.

To read the A2 sheet, you need to start on 3rd December 1960 and move along the lifeline found just above the timeline. Everything became confused after 18th December 2000, and it has taken me an awfully long time to sort my mind out and, as I said, it keeps on changing.

What is disconcerting is, I wrote the A2 equation backwards. I started with a yellow star with a question mark in the middle of an A4 piece of paper, whereas, logically, I should have started at the day of my birth and moved forward in time. So, I started at the centre of the universe – the exact centre of the pineal gland.

Each time I lift the red pen to edit this book, I learn more about the hidden meanings to my A2 equation and discover how they represent some of the many problems I have been facing. Often it is a case of simply getting the depictions in the right order!

For example, the spiritual stag is the head of all the animals in the forest; he's got his nose into everything, even over the barbed wire fence. He's the main man!

Then there's the messenger who holds the olive branch of peace that passes through the lightning! Nothing crosses the lightning!

However, I'm nowhere near understanding the hundreds of stories on this one A2 sheet – it is one hell of an equation or exploration of my distressed mind.

What I guess I'm trying to say is that it is confusing now and I will compromise. I'm putting this book together with what I have now and accepting that tomorrow it could all be different again.

IN THE TWILIGHT ZONE

After being operational for nearly 20 years, Fire Brigade Union member Mick Crowe fell mentally ill. Here's his story and how the Union helped him through it.

I am sure you have heard of the twilight zone. Well, I am going to tell you what it's like and how the FBU helped me to escape from it.

After being an operational firefighter for nearly 20 years I fell ill, mentally ill. At first, I got little understanding from my brigade. Then, I made a serious suicide attempt on my life, surviving by sheer luck.

Suffering from severe occupational and personal stress and from depression for some eleven months, I finally went out for lunch. Unbeknown to the police who attended my suicide attempt, I had already disposed of my shotguns. But

they still responded to my house with an armed response unit in scenes similar to the 1970s hit series The Sweeney. Obviously, they cannot be criticised for such action. After all, there are a lot of 'nutters' around!

The arrest — I was escorted to a jail cell by four or five police officers — wasn't too pleasant either. Although looking back, I do have to smile at the image of them as, having released my handcuffs, they all tried to get through a single door opening at the same time.

That was the beginning of perhaps a six-hour wait for my psychiatrist that would lead to me being sectioned under the Mental Health Act for 28 days and my 'voluntary' stay in a mental hospital for a further three and a half months. Thanks to illness and medication my memory of this experience is a bit hazy. But what I can recall from my incarceration was that I was supervised 24/7, walked on

THE PSYCHOTIC FIREMAN

the tables, spat my medication out and was totally psychotic and paranoid. On top of all that, the FBI was waiting outside ready to deport me in a UFO. "What a crazy world, eh!"

Well, I supposed you are wondering why I am telling you all of this personal stuff? The fact is my illness was genuine. So why was it not taken seriously from day one when I handed in my sick- note? It did appear that some in management knew more than my doctors, although they have never seen my medical records (they are some inches thick by now!).

The real nitty-gritty stuff came to light when I was retired from the job. After speaking to my doctors, I applied for a qualifying injury award because they believed a significant proportion of my illness was attributed to my operational duties. Although doctors do not like to label anyone with a mental illness, post-traumatic

stress-disorder, psychotic depression and schizophrenia were all mentioned early on. Easy you might think, pension him off and retire him. But it was not so simple.

In all, it took the Shropshire Fire and Rescue Service and in particular Mike, former Shropshire FBU brigade secretary, four years to settle the claim. Mike spent countless hours on this case, fighting for my cause at a time when I was too unwell to fend for myself. Once the award was granted, the brigade still dragged its feet – at a time when I could have done with the settlement from a financial point of view but also for my mental wellbeing. The brigade took it right up to the point where they were threatened with legal action.

Towards the end, Mike and the brigade arranged an advance on my injury award relating to the minimum amount I would receive in any event, prior to a final settlement being agreed.

Apparently, this is ground-breaking and well worth noting for the future.

STANDING ON A TABLE

In 20 years, I have never needed the FBU. But they were there when I finally needed them. I can remember standing on a table in hospital moaning at Mike and the occupational nurse, Caroline (somebody else I thought I would never need) that they had taken my belt away. I pulled my trousers down over my hips to show them how much weight I had lost and that I could not keep my trousers up. Unfortunately, they could not sort that one out for me! Through loyalty, Mike continued with my case even after his retirement, as did my psychiatrist. So, this world does still have nice people!

My final words of advice are these: value your FBU because you never know when you need it; marry a good wife to help you through the bad times; never take things too seriously and never, ever, lose your sense of humour. After what 'we' went through, if you cannot laugh about it you will surely go nuts!

FBU COMMENT

We had a difficult time representing Mick Crowe. It was decided to allow our retiring brigade secretary (2003) to continue his close working relationship with our member. The Brigade Committee and I wish to thank Samuel, formerly of Thompson's solicitors, for his advice. But very special thanks and well done to Mike Who never gave up and achieved a successful outcome for our member. Our member is well on the road to recovery and is rebuilding his life with his loving and supportive wife and family.

Tom
FBU Brigade Secretary, Shropshire

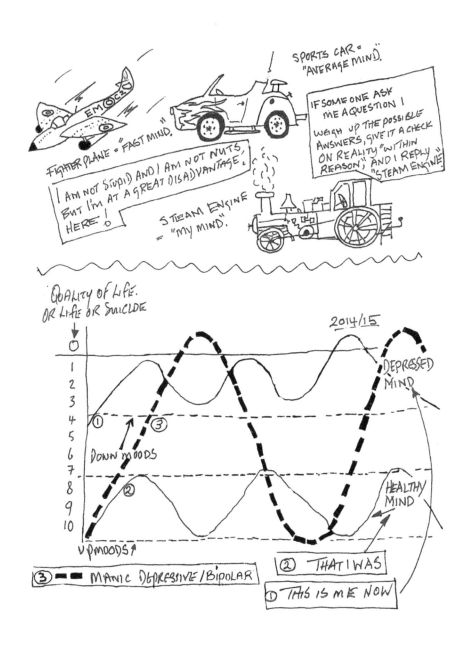

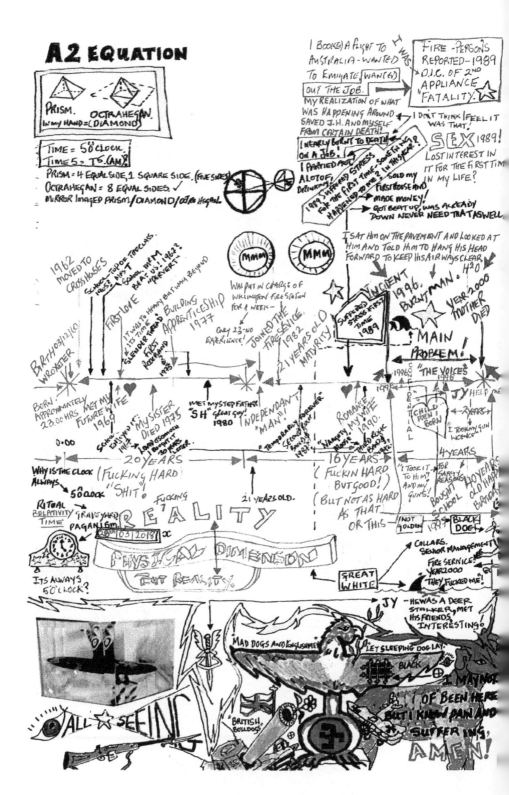

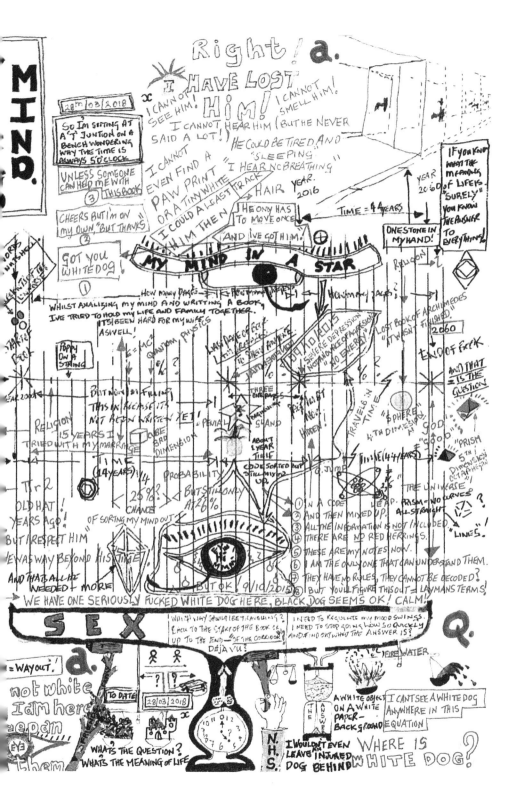

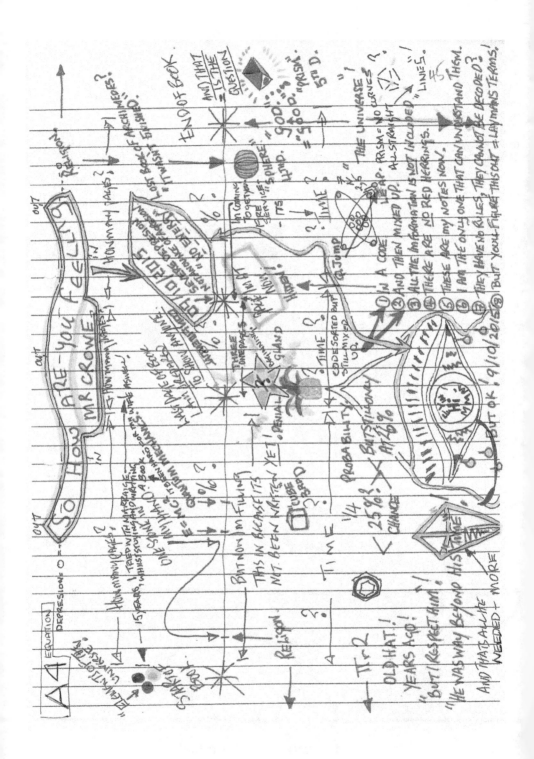

YOU COME TO A 'T' JUNCTION ON THE ROAD
WHERE THERE ARE TWO BROTHERS, Ⓐ+Ⓑ.
ONE ALWAYS TELLS LIES AND THE OTHER
ALWAYS TELLS THE TRUTH.
THE **DARK** AND THE LIGHT,
THE **BLACK** AND THE WHITE.
YOU NEED TO ASK WHICH WAY IS THE
NEAREST TOWN.
YOU CAN ONLY ASK ONE QUESTION TO
ONE BROTHER, WHAT IS THE QUESTION
YOU ASK HIM?

THAT IS THE QUESTION.

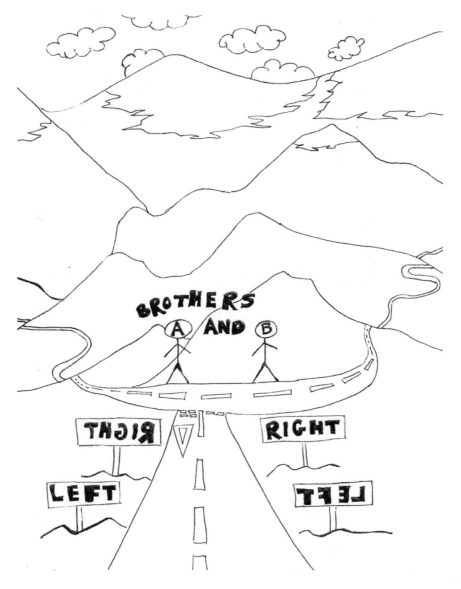

T-junction

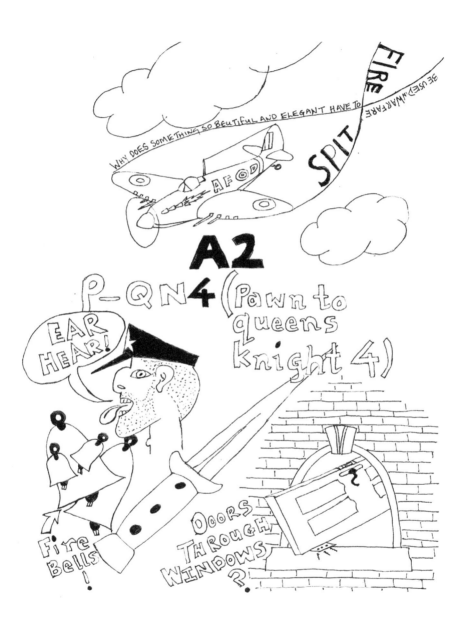

CHAPTER 6

The Big Bang

You can see from my jottings that something happened in my mind at the start of the new millennium. Apart from being seriously ill, my mind was finding loads of locked away memories. I had opened doorways in my mind, but with these memories came information, knowledge, questions, and answers. I felt as if I knew everything; that my mind was capable of anything. My mind was in overdrive. Sadly, though, it is now burned out – and that is who I am today.

I came up with a lot of theories and then analysed them, and I think I sometimes got them right. I believe my door to the subconscious opened wide and I could see inside, and I now know how that door was opened.

It was an early morning shout in 1996 and we attended a person's reported house fire. When we arrived, I was told a mother and two children were trapped upstairs. We could see the flames had engulfed downstairs and were rapidly spreading up to the next floor. The officer in charge, Mike, ordered the two lads with breathing apparatus into the building.

I heard a loud, constant groaning from a police car while I was operating the pump, only to see a severely burned man sitting in the back seat. I ran over, got him out and told him to sit on the kerb by the fire appliance. His eyes were transfixed on me with an overpowering stare, pleading for help. We were later told he had re-entered the lounge and attempted to carry out a burning armchair, only to get trapped with it in the hallway causing the fire to escalate straight up the stairs, accelerated by flammable paints under the staircase.

I crouched down in front of him and looked at him. I told him to hang his head forward and keep his airways clear, then I put his hands in a bucket of water and sprayed him with water from the hose reel.

That's when it happened.

The burned man I sprayed with water in 1996 and my mother's deathbed groan were identical but for exactly the opposite reasons. The man's moan was in relief at the cooling effect of the water, but my mother's was in pain. It took me a long time to remember back to the incident in 1996, over twenty years in fact, but my mother brought it back to me four years later after the event took place. It stirred up a hornet's nest and messed up my head.

The lads from work were great and they even found me a newspaper cutting about it. Eventually, I could remember more, like considering doing a tracheotomy on the man if his airways had closed-up, but I had never been trained for such a procedure and was worried about nicking an artery. Could you imagine the bloody scene?

When the second appliance turned up, and I handed the hose over, I remember shouting to them to feel the water constantly since it might get hot as the pump was getting warm. I remember looking at one child in the back of the ambulance: he was severely burned and shaking, and when he looked directly at me, I smiled, even though there was nothing to smile about.

Although it was an early morning shout, it felt like it was already night-time. Everything was dark around me. A newspaper article that night suggested the child was deemed critical; we took flowers to the grandmother living opposite the next day, and we could tell she appreciated our visit.

Well, if you've got this far, I've captured your attention. So let me detail my theory about the big bang. Yes – the big bang! Bear with me since the proposition came to me whilst sitting in a hospital waiting room (3682 words in a nutshell).

So here goes:

Have you ever wondered why the planets are spheres? Well, my theory is this: all the planets were a closely connected cluster of rocks, slowly spinning and gathering speed. Eventually, because of the heat being generated, there was a colossal explosion – a big bang – and our solar system was born. Gravity, magnetism, temperature and many other elements caused this spinning, leading to the birth of the sun and pushing the planets away.

Our universe, "the real big bang", will keep expanding until there is no more momentum from the effects of that first colossal event. When this happens, it will contract, or it will stand still in dormant space. That will be the end of our universe; beyond it is only space, and time no longer exists.

That is the beginning of the universe as we know it, but maybe not the end. Imagine another big bang elsewhere, creating another universe? This parallel universe will expand and maybe reach our own universe, causing gravitational and magnetic pulls again, so in fact it is a chain reaction. Understand this: everything in every direction is infinite. I'm afraid you need to understand the planets have always been there in some shape or form and always will be, but they will be forever changing into the next cycle. Obviously, the earth will eventually die, so to survive we need to move on.

Some people believe in God, they even pray to him, along with everything else which goes with that belief. I believe in an almighty power and I have the evidence in my head to prove it. We are connected to this almighty power and so we are all connected. It is a large network; everything which lives must die and we are all in it together. We go back to the elements and are born from the elements, and the pineal gland is the main connection between the physical and metaphysical, or spiritual, worlds.

It is meant to be an enlightenment when your pineal gland opens – it is like a third eye. So what went wrong with me, then? My third eye opened whilst I was waiting in a hospital waiting room, sitting opposite the severely burned man I've told you about. He kept staring at me, transfixed. How could he be sitting there four years after the event? I covered my face with my hands to stop him staring at me and that's when it happened. My head went on fire, with blisters bubbling from my cheeks and forehead like when I found the burning body I'd stepped on.

I believe very little is known about this organ at the centre of the brain, so what I suggest now may be disputed. It's difficult to segregate science and spirituality because they work hand-in-hand. I'm afraid I will not refer to it as God, though you may if you wish to. To me, it is an almighty power: 'the answer to everything'.

I believe I was using a very large proportion of my brain power during my experience but I was extremely ill with it. Impossible, you may say, when the average person only uses about 20%, but I did, possibly using even more than 75%. I could see other dimensions and I believe I travelled in the fourth of these and even travelled in time. The past is easier, but the future is more difficult to see. Sometimes, I feel I could travel again if I stopped my medication, but it helps in this 'third dimension' which is where I am now.

I suggest you research 'near-death experiences', 'outer body experiences', 'remote viewing', 'telepathy' and 'time travel' because I'm not going to write about things people have already written about. I also believe that ancient and lost civilisations knew more than us, and I've experienced it all too.

My psychiatrist once asked me if I thought I could read people's minds or if they could read mine, and my answer was this: "If I could read your mind you need not have asked me the question and if you could read mine, I would have no need to give you an answer."

Is this strictly right, though? What if I already knew what he would ask and had the answer before he asked the question? Think about it.

You have probably heard of *The God Particle* (by Leon M Lederman and Dick Teresi) but what about the spirit molecule dimethyltryptamine (DMT)? I believe large amounts of this are released at birth and death, but my mind died at forty, so I was probably overloaded with this in midlife. What effect would that have on my mind? I know it has been linked with psychedelic experiences. Maybe this caused my psychosis?

I believe my illness damaged my brain, so I used another part of it. The original part I was using is still functioning, but now I also have a new area which is working. These parts don't work properly together and the main man, the pineal gland, can't sort them out.

I'm in a state of confusion at times. I quote: 'the pineal gland connects the soul system with the nervous system, and it converts the sympathetic nerve signals to the main nervous system'. At least, it did in my network, and when this happened, I developed body shakes. A tricky little gland, I would say; it allows me to function in this world but also allows me to see into others, like something out of science fiction.

I have endeavoured to show the workings of my mind and what went wrong in the A2 equation. But, like I've said before, I didn't know what I was writing when I wrote it; sometimes my hand just does its own thing without me thinking about it. I don't know where it comes from, but my only explanation is the pineal gland, the soul, my innermost thoughts.

Maybe all of this is just in my mind, but if you can't believe your own mind, what can you believe? Nobody can explain how memory works, but I can explain how I believe it works. When someone has a good memory or is having flashbacks, I would call it 'time travel in the mind'. Recalling a memory, something which has already happened, is travelling back in time. People with excellent memories travel better – and if you can travel backwards, why not travel forward?

So I reckon I questioned what life was all about when I tried to commit suicide – the *ultimate question*. I looked for the answer in my head and it's all in the mind – *the answer to everything*. I had no choice but to try to kill myself as my third eye opened and with it came knowledge and insight into different realms I hadn't visited before. The amount of information to be analysed is astronomical and if one person manages to sort the answer to everything, they should keep it to themselves – *otherwise, it would be the end of mankind*.

I have seen unbelievable things in this world, but I have been to different realms and seen unbelievable things there too. I am not mad; I just believe what I witnessed happened, and there's no doubt I'm different because of my experience.

Articles in magazines and newspapers over the years helped verify my view, but they are basic and hardly scrape the surface. I quote: 'the eventual goal of science is to provide a single theory which describes the whole universe', but to date they can't crack it. However, I hope you have gained something from my contribution to this big question.

I first put pen to paper to tell my doctor what was going on in my head; that writing has now become this book. Through it, I hope you have gained some insight into my attempt to sort this knackered computer out in my head without a bloody manual to help.

(NOTES) 4TH DIMENSION = A SPHERE

IMAGINE you ARE FLOATING IN A DARK ROOM, EXACTLY
IN THE DEAD CENTRE OF IT! LETS GET MORE EXACT,
LETS PLACE THE DEAD CENTRE OF THE PENIAL GLAND
IN THE CENTRE OF THE UNIVERSE / ROOM, OR SAY THE
CENTRE OF A SPHERE.

AN EQUAL DISTANCE
IN EVERY
DIRECTION.
FROM THE CENTRE
OF THE UNIVERSE

SPHERE

PENIAL GLAND

SPACE

BECAUSE IT IS DARK AND YOU CAN'T SEE ANYTHING EVERY
DIRECTION IS INFINATE AND you ARE THE CENTRE OF
THE UNIVERSE, ITS NOT AN AREA OR PLANET, IT IS YOU,
TO A PIN HEAD SIZE, NOW you CAN'T GET MORE
EXACT THAN THAT CONSIDERING THE SIZE OF THE
UNIVERSE!
        RENE DESCARTES SAID "THE PENIAL GLAND IS THE PRINCIPLE-"
"SEAT OF THE SOUL" (THE ANTENNA TO THE UNIVERSE.)
"IT IS ACTUALLY" ➔ (THE CENTRE OF THE UNIVERSE.)

(NOTES)

5TH DIMENSION = A PRISM.

RED BLUE
YELLOW

LIGHT / OPICAL / RAINBOW?
COLOURS

DIAMOND?

NOW I DON'T HAVE A FUCKIN CLUE ON WHAT I'VE JUST DONE!
OR WRITTEN

REFRACTION

PRIME COLOURS? RAINBOW? LIGHT?
"BUT I CAN'T SORT THIS FUCKER AT THE MOMENT"?
I THINK ILL PUT IT IN NOTES OF THE BOOK!

FUCK ME, BENDING LIGHT / TIME,
DEVIATION ANGLES AND DISPERSION ——— ANGLE OF INCIDENCE?

$$\delta_1' = \arcsin \left| \frac{n_0}{n_1} \sin \delta_0 \right|$$

" I AIN'T GOT A CLUE WHAT THAT MEANS"!

"TOO MUCH FOR FUCKIN ME"!

& TIME

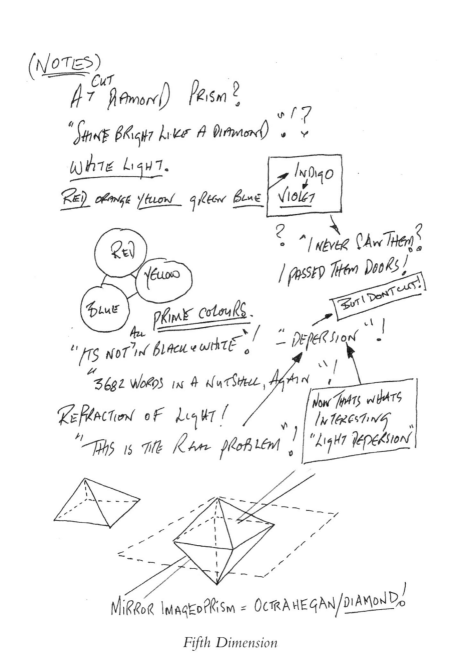

Fifth Dimension

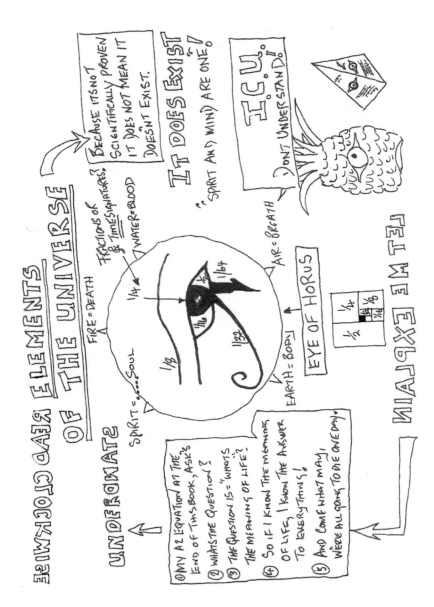

Elements of the Universe

POSTSCRIPT

As you have just read, I wrote this book so people can learn from it, at the very least. If they do, then my illness has served some purpose. It's not fair that anyone should go through what I have, but believe me, illness can come on at any time and afflict any one of us.

My life became a total mess in 2000 and still is, to a great extent, but so did the lives of my wife and children – lives which will never be the same again. Enormous damage has been done to my family.

I have tried hard but, since 2000, everything has been and remains a struggle. When I came out of hospital, my wife and I somehow held the marriage together for another fourteen years. I could never properly interact with the kids since I was often lost in my own thoughts but we can both be proud that some good has come of it all in that we have two lovely, well- mannered girls.

My wife and I separated in 2014. Eighteen months later, we moved back in together, since we had become friends again in that time and the cost of running two houses was crippling us.

Although I didn't physically die, I mentally turned off and died in the mind I passed over when I saw and heard the crusher coming down in the bin wagon outside my house. Somehow, the doctors brought me back again into this world, but during that time I experienced something else – other dimensions. A near-death experience, some may call it.

I saw all the usual things but I can't tell you everything and that's the way it is. I'm afraid I was allowed back into this dimension with certain restrictions; I'm a man of my word and I promised not to divulge everything – you need not understand or know it all.

Wisdom is knowing you are not always right, but my three short stories were written for a reason and that is to help me find my way out of the labyrinth in my mind. They mean something; I just need to figure out the last short story. Figure out why the time is always five o'clock and what the screaming in my left ear is.

I've travelled around extensively in the fourth dimension and even stepped into the fifth for a while. The fourth is relatively understandable, but the fifth is a brain twister.

It appeared as something I recognised amongst masses of souls, upon masses and masses of souls on every horizon. It acknowledged me, though, and I knew it was not my time to go. I was blessed with life and I stepped back through the double doors and ended my journey. Apparently, I had not finished what I had to do in the third. That was the message I was given, but I'm struggling to find my way back to reality.

I can see into my mind. I can read it like a book, but I can't get it all in the right order so it's very confusing. I feel I can sort out the reality and psychosis, but it takes time, which is why I now struggle with stress.

All of it together is too much, therefore I need to step back from a normal life. I tried to explain to my doctors that my mind was like an elastic band: the more it is pulled and twisted, the easier it is to make it twang and break. I believe the doctors don't have an effective enough superglue to fix it. The elastic band is still there in one piece, but it doesn't do its job anymore. Maybe a glue will be found one day, or maybe not. I just hope something can be found for future generations.

Writing this book wasn't easy. The stress in so doing could have killed me. It could get me locked up. It could make me a famous writer (but then again, maybe not!).

But it could also help make me well again and perhaps help others.

So you see, the book is my mind, and so my mind is this book! When I refer to my book, I'm also referring to my mind. I hope you get the picture?

We come from the universe, and we go back into it.

A DAUGHTER'S ADDITION

I am the eldest of Mick's two 'well- mannered' daughters as he has described us. For many reasons, he asked me to reorganise and make the first edit of this book to the best of my ability. I'd like to think, and hope, I've done it justice, especially being a budding writer myself. He also asked me to add a brief note at the end, and here it is.

While I was editing this, my grandfather passed away – the grandfather on my father's side who has been mentioned several times throughout this book. Unfortunately, I can't remember my father's mother nor his step-father, but reading this book, I can't help but think that's for the best!

One evening, my father came into the room, announcing he had some 'bad news' for me. "Oh no, what is it?" was my response, because there aren't many things which I thought could go wrong at that moment.

"The police were just here," was what he started with, and naturally my stomach dropped. What had the police wanted here? "They've found grandad, and he's died."

My first response was to get up and hug him because that's the natural reaction anyone would have. I gave him a tight squeeze and yet I had mixed emotions, and I didn't cry at first. My grandfather had visited us a lot when I was a child, but those visits became less as I grew older, so I didn't really feel attached to him anymore. I didn't feel that upset, especially having read what he was like to my father when he was a child. But the death of a person makes you question things. *Could I have done more? Did they know I loved them? When did I see them last? Did we last separate on a friendly note?*

That didn't stop me from being the one who cried the most at his funeral. Whether it was because the thought of death scares me (never being able to see that person alive again, you know?) or because thoughts of him came flooding back, I couldn't say. All I know is that love is a funny thing and people show it in many different ways, but as we change, so does our way of showing love.

My father mentioned he'd called his father the night before his death and set his mind at rest when my grandfather threw a barrage of questions at him – about the mistakes he'd made. Could they be forgiven? My father said everyone makes mistakes, and he'd made some himself, it's just life. It's not hard to believe my grandfather now felt he could move on and just let go. In a case like that, death almost seems like it's an option for the dying. My mother always says you should part with any person as if it's the last time you'll see them alive, because you don't know what life and the future will bring.

Reading this book as a writer myself made me wish I could come up with such bizarre yet logical stories (*One Stone in My Hand* is where I felt this most strongly).

Reading this book as a daughter made me understand so much more about my father and my family's life before I could remember it.

Reading this book as a human raised questions I didn't know I had, answered things I didn't know I needed or wanted answers to. But I think, most importantly, it made me see all kinds of things from a fresh angle.

My father didn't want to touch this book after he'd written it, or to add anything else which has happened since its creation, so I felt I should add the bit about my grandfather. His death happened at a bit of a turning point in my own life, and a turning point in the life of the world. As I write, Covid- 19 is ravaging the world; I finished editing this book during the England lockdown on 27th March 2020.

Much like my father doesn't believe he'll be the same again after his mental illness, I don't believe the world will be the same after this viral illness. I want to take this last line to say that much like my father survived with the help of others, we should remember that others need kindness, not only in the last and darkest moments of their lives, but at all times.

WELL, I NEVER EXPECTED THAT EITHER! – A WIFE'S ADDITION

Mick's most vivid memory from when he and I got together was me reading all the time. My nose could easily be stuck in a book all day. As soon as I got my pocket money, I would spend it on buying a book and sit in my room all day to read it! I love books – I can read anything, even the most boring stuff, hoping that it might get better – and to find out whether it did in the end. It is the reading itself that gives me pleasure.

Yet, it took me a lot to read Mick's book.

It started at some point during his illness and I can still remember him writing it; it fills me with deepest sorrow and upset. It was then that I knew something was seriously wrong with him - but I never even envisaged in the slightest just *how much* was actually wrong with him. Mick was never the academic type. Saying that he is by no means stupid, lazy or lacking ambition. But he wouldn't read or learn something simply for the joy of it – unless it was a practical skill.

So there we were: Mick, in the becoming of a published author writing his first (and most likely only) book, and me, watching him writing the first (and maybe only) book I did not fancy reading. This book took a tremendous toll on me when he wrote it. He would sit there at the kitchen table, unshaven and unwashed with greasy hair and filthy clothes and write with such vigour that the whole kitchen table would shake. He did this for hours, day and night, drinking brandy and hardly sleeping apart from the odd hour at the kitchen table. Writing, writing, writing. And this wasn't going on for days, but for weeks – maybe even months. And yet, no one else noticed that he was ill at all. People were wondering what was wrong with him, if anything at all, and his doctor was oblivious to it as well. Mick was a champ in hiding it!

Before Mick fell mentally ill, I never had much patience for people with poor mental health. Back then, my opinion had been that they just needed to get their act together. And their family? It never crossed my mind they would be affected so much. Since then, however, I know that it is not that easy. Mick's illness taught me that there is no easy fix. His illness taught me that people with poor mental health need a lot of support and understanding and to not be judged so quickly. I now understand they don't want to take their medication. They cannot necessarily see they are ill, never mind *how* ill they are. The world they live in is *real* for them! In their opinion, it is *we* who don't have a clue and insight into what is *really* going on! It is we, the healthy minds, who are actually in need of correction! I don't want to count up all the minor and major incidents that happened during his illness, but I will share one incident that visualised this distortion of the world he lived in very vividly.

One day, we all went to the shopping center in Telford. It was dark early, and it was a very miserable day: windy, wet and cold. Mick was already on medication but by no means out of the pit yet. As we drove along, a leaf blew over the road, and I shouted out: 'Oh, look, a mouse!', to which Mick replied, 'No, that was a leaf'. I agreed as it made more sense, and besides, its movement was floating rather than running. However, Mick then insisted that it was a mouse which turned into a leaf! When I explained to him that wasn't possible and it was most likely me being mistaken for the reasons just mentioned, he kept quiet. About 15 minutes later, he said to me: 'You were right; a mouse can't turn into a leaf'. It took him all that time to work out the obvious. For me, the subject was closed, obviously. For him, it remained a misery and only because he figured out the reality could I catch a glimpse into his twisted mind which was still a long way away from being healed.

When Mick fell ill, he became a different person. He changed so much that I didn't recognise him anymore. The man who had once been one of the most caring, reliable and loving people I had ever known and who had been worshipping me not too long ago became a horrible, ignorant and aggressive person. He started to scare me and the girls to the point that we all slept in Danny's bedroom; I had to put a wedge under the door and barricade it, so we felt safe. He did and said things that weren't him – they came from this monster which had taken over and made him do these horrible things. If it hadn't been for knowing him nearly all my life and knowing that he had no one else but me looking out for him, I would have left him. I would have gone somewhere else to keep us all safe. How many other people are putting up being ill-treated and yet stick it out to be there for a loved one? How many husbands, wives, mothers, fathers, siblings and friends? And hardly anyone understands, never mind emphasises what *they* go through. For me, the only option was to go back to Germany, leaving the love of my life behind, knowing he would be lost to this monster, and God knows if he really would end up a nutcase at Shelton Mental Hospital for the rest of his life. How many people are in the same position and are asked, 'Well, why don't you leave him?', I am sure the answer is much more complex than people anticipate most of the time. It's no good asking the question – unless a structured support frame is offered at the same time. If you can't offer this first, just don't ask the question; it's more destroying than helpful!

Many things have luckily changed since Mick fell ill, and society has become much more aware and supportive of mental health issues, but this is still only touching the tip of the iceberg. You can simply not fathom something you haven't experienced first-hand. You can only get some (vague) idea. And this is the reason why I, too, am adding something to this book. To emphasize that mentally ill people need all the help, understanding and empathy we can offer. To let people know it is worth it to keep fighting, whether being ill themselves or looking after someone mentally unwell. To advise people to not take doctors' words for granted. They are right in most cases, and I would expect the GPs and psychiatrists to seek permission from their patients to involve the partner in all of their decisions. After all, it is you - the partner, the parent, the guardian - who know the patient best! You know how well - or little - the medication works. You know first about the solutions or problems that come along with the therapy. It is you, who can and *should* advise the professionals to shed that little bit more clarity on the treatment, the parts they cannot see. Even when Mick was under 24/7 supervision, he needed *my* input to improve. The nurses and the psychiatrist needed *my* input to understand better if and how well his medication was working. You are the voice of the person who is caught up in their own space and time, far away from everybody else's.

The anecdotes I could talk about are unbelievable. Surreal. Nobody knew about this as I had no one to talk to — and besides: what difference would that have made? I went to the doctor and begged him for help - I was in tears, but no help was offered. But frankly? I think he was out of his depth. He was not trained enough to understand mental health issues. This is no complaint about his skills as a doctor; he had been a great doctor, and we stayed with him afterwards until he retired. But he just didn't read the signs – and only when I refused to leave his office with my two little children did he finally agree to refer Mick to a psychiatrist. I should have insisted much earlier – it was almost too late by then. Why I didn't? Well, you don't want to be a pain, you don't feel right questioning the expert's expertise, and you have hope: that it *will* get better. Mick nearly paid with his life because I was dithering; I nearly lost my husband, and the girls nearly lost their dad. But I don't blame myself for this. I did what I could under the given circumstances. I couldn't have done better, and I couldn't have tried harder. So there is no blame to take but to count my blessings that it was just about working out for us.

Still, in hindsight, I should have been persistent much sooner. Even the most expertly experts are allowed to make mistakes since they too are only human, after all. *If* there had been anyone to blame, I would have to be blamed just the same for not being more persistent as soon as I realized something was seriously wrong. Now, knowing more about paranoia and schizophrenia, the signs were all too clear. At the beginning of Mick's journey to recovery, I would spot the signs immediately and could tell when Mick hadn't taken his medication. I could tell when the dosage of his medication had been changed. What worked well and what didn't even before he would notice himself. Like so many other mentally unwell people, Mick had to come to terms with the fact that he depends on medication to stay well. This process took years, and I am incredibly proud of him that he finally accepted it. This significant step of acceptance has made our lives easier and more enjoyable; it has allowed him to become a better father and husband again. Getting to this stage is a constant battle for the mentally ill.

First, they have to acknowledge that something is wrong with them. Easier said than done when you are living in your own little disillusioned world. When they take their medication, they feel the world around them changes again. They get better, and for some reason they think they don't need their medicine anymore. They may keep forgetting because they feel well. And hey, who wants to be paranoid, schizophrenic, depressed or mentally ill altogether? It is still stigmatized – yes, much less so, but it still is. Mick's main argument was that he didn't want to take his medicine for the rest of his life because of the side effects. I reminded him that a family member of ours has had to take medication since she was three because of her kidneys. The side effects are so worrying that whenever she went for a sleepover, even as a teenager, I asked the parents to look after her medication to prevent a child from taking them by accident. I asked him how he would feel if I decided she should no longer take it since she is doing okay at the moment, especially since the side effects are so worrying. I think this was one of the main points that made him think and reconsider. But it was a long way until he was in a fit enough state to take this in. We had so many ups and downs when he didn't take his meds. He would forget, and because he still felt well the next day, the next, and the next – well, what's the point in taking it? The point is that the medicine isn't out of the system with a bang. Its effect goes slowly, and the madness retakes its place slowly and cunningly, so the patient doesn't notice. But the loved ones do. And I couldn't count the times I asked Mick when he took his last medication. We had arguments over it, but luckily he realized fairly soon that they *must* work in some way if I would notice that he hadn't taken it.

Today, we count our blessings. It could always be worse, and there is always some good in everything. You only need to look hard enough, and sometimes you don't realise until a long time has passed. Mick is reasonably well today; at least, he functions normally most of the time! Today, he is a loving father and caring husband. He still has his ups and downs though, and to be frank it *can* be frustrating at times, but then I think about how frustrating it must feel for him. Sometimes, life is a struggle for him. He tries to keep it away from me and the girls, and he is grateful for having his family around him. But it is a struggle nonetheless, and we often forget that mentally ill people have to fight every day not to get drowned by their sorrows, knowing that this will never change. Life can be made more manageable, like giving a paralysed person a wheelchair – but it is still not the same as being your healthy self. All that is left is that we count our blessings and are grateful for what we have got – not being miserable about what we *haven't* got!

EDITOR'S POSTSCRIPT

It has taken Mick nearly 4 years to get this book to a stage where it is publishable. At times, he couldn't lift his hands off the desk and onto the keyboard. Indeed, each painstakingly slow step has taken a gritty mix of angst and plenty of sweat and tears.

Throughout all his deeply difficult times, Mick remains a fervent support of the fire and other emergency services. Times have changed, and he hopes that his book does not cause offence, but, forty years ago, things were done differently.

He has met some wonderful people, made some great friends and is pleased and proud to have served and protected a small part of our nation.

However, each difficult word he's typed has been therapeutic: huge, black clouds of depression have lifted from his mind and his persona is brighter, simply by being able to get this tale out and written down on paper.

By no means is Mick a well man, but he now sees things more clearly and he increasingly finds times where he is in a better, calmer place. He accepts, though, that he's living with a huge black dog on his back that he'll never shake off.

Importantly though, his wife and two daughters have benefitted greatly from reading these words. They are now travelling with him on his journey with a better understanding of where the man they loved went to and what he is still suffering.

Lightning Source UK Ltd.
Milton Keynes UK
UKHW041256050123
414884UK00001B/17